ALSO BY CASEY MEYERS

Aerobic Walking

Walking

Casey Meyers

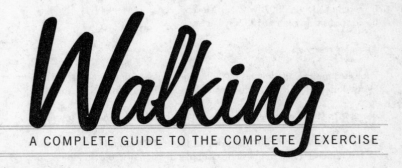

Walking

A COMPLETE GUIDE TO THE COMPLETE EXERCISE

BALLANTINE BOOKS

New York

2007 Ballantine Books Trade Paperback Edition

Published in the United States by Ballantine Books, an imprint of The Random House Publishing Group, a division of Random House, Inc., New York.

BALLANTINE and colophon are registered trademarks of Random House, Inc.

Originally published in different form in 1992 by Random House, an imprint of The Random House Publishing Group, a division of Random House, Inc.

LIBRARY OF CONGRESS CATALOGING-IN-PUBLICATION DATA
Meyers, Casey.
    Walking : a complete guide to the complete exercise / Casey Meyers.
        p. cm.
    A revision of the 1st ed., New York : Random House, 1992.
    Includes bibliographical references and index.
    ISBN 978-0-345-49104-6
    1. Walking. 2. Exercise. I. Title.
    GV502.M49 2007   613.7'17—dc22   2006042878

Printed in the United States of America

www.ballantinebooks.com

9 8 7 6 5 4 3 2 1

Book design by Casey Hampton

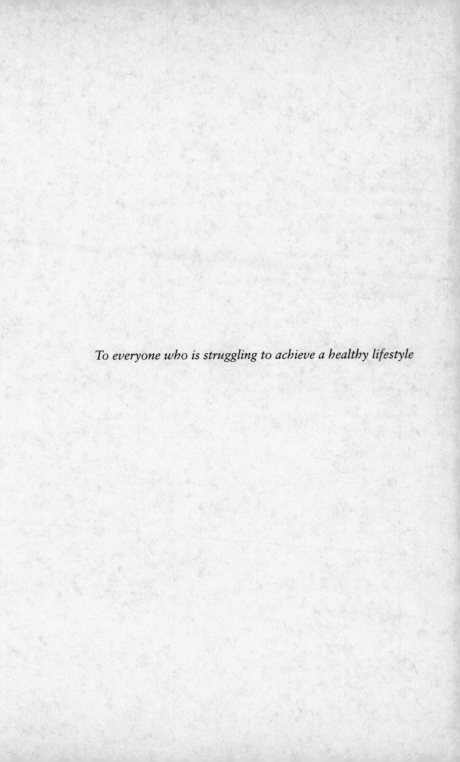

To everyone who is struggling to achieve a healthy lifestyle

The sovereign invigorator of the body is exercise, and of all the exercises, walking is best.

—THOMAS JEFFERSON

GEORGE SHEEHAN, M.D.

Foreword

Our beach house on the Jersey Shore overlooks a boardwalk that extends for a mile to the north and five miles to the south. All year long when the weather is right, walkers and runners and cyclists pass by.

The walkers are by far the most numerous. Some are solitary, deep in thought or gazing at the surf and the sea gulls. Others are in groups, couples in quiet conversation or threesomes talking animatedly. Still others are engaged in earnest effort, arms bent at the elbow and swinging to a rapid cadence. All are experiencing the benefits and the pleasures of walking.

What is happening on our boardwalk is happening all over the country. There has been a renaissance in walking. Walkers are rediscovering what has been known over the centuries. Walking has a global effect on the entire person. It adds hours to one's day and years to one's life. Walking is a superior way to handle stress and provides the isolation needed for meditation. Not the least of its benefits is the opportunity it gives for creative thinking and solving life's problems.

If these rewards seem similar to the claims made by runners and cyclists and adherents of other activities, it is because they are. Exercise is the generic drug. Walking and running and cycling are simply brands, of which there are many, and all equally effective.

Watching these enthusiasts pass by, I am reminded of the comment Dr. Elliot Joslin, the legendary diabetic specialist, made when asked what the best form of insulin was. "All insulins are good insulins if you know how to use them." This is certainly true about exercise. All exercises are good exercises if you know how to use them. And of all these exercises, walking has the longest history, the best pedigree, the most distinguished practitioners. Walking was Nature's first exercise, and has been recommended by authorities over the centuries.

In the first book totally devoted to exercise, published in 1555, Cristóbal Méndez writes: "The best and most beneficial exercise is walking." Méndez gives many reasons for selecting walking. It fulfills all the requirements and is so easy that no matter where you are you can do it. Even more important, according to Méndez, walking offers many pleasures and joys. He points out that you can observe, read, converse, sing, meditate, and practice all your mental skills such as imagination, cogitation, and memory.

Harry Andrews, the most highly respected track coach at the turn of the century, was another proponent of walking. Andrews included among his athletes Walter George, the world's best at the mile, and the incomparable Alfie Shrubb, who once held all the world's records for distances from 2 miles to 15 miles, and many other runners, boxers, and cyclists of the time.

Andrews regarded walking as fundamental to all training. "Experience tells me," he writes, "that walking should represent the groundwork for any system of training." It did not matter to him what sport you were in, whether running, boxing, fencing, cycling, or rowing; walking as a primary exercise was applicable to all. According to Andrews, "It gave by far the greatest benefit of any form of training in its result."

For those interested only in fitness, walking was his recommended activity. He saw no need to do anything else. It was a superior way to reduce weight and there was no need to worry about pace. "The best advice I can give," he wrote, "is to make your own pace—the pace, in fact, that will suit you best. This pace will almost certainly be an average of four miles an hour."

In the lines above I have presented evidence from the distant past. In this book Casey Meyers brings us up to date on research, both his own and that of others, proving that walking is for everybody. The overweight, out-of-shape beginner, the accomplished athlete, and everyone in between will benefit by making walking part of their lives.

Preface

I clearly remember the morning of May 14, 1999. I was having a coronary angiogram in the cardiac unit of Heartland Regional Medical Center in St. Joseph, Missouri, where I live. To test my awareness, Dr. Steven Rowe, my cardiologist, leaned in close to my face and in a loud voice said, "Casey, do you know who this is?" I blinked a couple of times to clear away the fog that my mind was in from the heavy sedation and muttered, "Yeah, it's Dr. Rowe." He then said, "You've got massive blockage in your main artery. The left anterior descending artery is ninety-nine percent closed." His chilling diagnosis was, "This is life-threatening, and I can't let you off of the table until it is repaired." I have since learned that the medical profession frequently refers to this artery as the "widow maker," because blockage in that artery is often fatal.

I am writing this updated version of *Walking* at the age of 79. I have been listed as "high risk" for heart attack or stroke for over ten years, and so far I've had neither. I believe I am still enjoying a full life primarily because of an active lifestyle, a heart-healthy diet, and my daily 3-mile walks. Every morning I am out early, walking for my life—literally.

The first indication that I had a heart problem occurred in November 1995 at the prestigious Cooper Clinic in Dallas, Texas, run by Dr. Kenneth Cooper, author of the revolutionary exercise book *Aerobics* in 1968, and a pioneer in preventative medicine since 1970. I have had an annual physical there for over twenty years. Because of my age (I was 67 at the time), my doctor thought that I should have a CT scan of my heart even though I always tested at a superior level on the treadmill stress test. I was stunned when the scan revealed that I had extensive calcium deposits in my coronary arteries, especially the left anterior descending artery. The report stated, "He has a *very high* probability of flow-obstructing (functional) disease." My calcium score was 1,168, and the chart only went to 1,200. The next week I had a thallium heart scan at the Cooper Clinic to determine if the blockage was severe enough to warrant an invasive procedure. The scan involved injecting dye into the bloodstream, stressing the body on a treadmill, and then measuring the blood flow in the heart on a nuclear scanner. This procedure revealed only mild disease, and because of my high fitness level, no symptoms, and no other risk factors other than age, the doctor decided to continue monitoring my heart. A 1997 CT scan showed a "low rate of progression" compared to 1995, and so monitoring continued.

In October 1998 I was 70 years old and once again tested superior on my treadmill stress test. For this stress test, I had trained to where I could walk 5 miles in 58 minutes. Several years earlier, because of arthritis, I had to have a total replacement of my right knee. The Cooper Clinic has the largest data base of treadmill testing on the relationship between fitness and health in the world. No 70-year-old—or anyone of any age—had ever tested superior with an artificial knee before. My personal goal was to be the first (and maybe the last). I was truly elated that I was able to do it, but my elation was short-lived.

The results of the stress test were equivocal, revealing there were some minor EKG changes noted near peak exercise and occasional premature beats noted during the recovery phase. The results were not alarming, but in light of the extensive calcium deposits in my coronary arteries, my doctor felt we should do another thallium scan on my next physical, using their advanced scanning technology. I opted to do it sooner, but since there seemed to be no urgency I waited until after quail and pheasant season in Missouri and Kansas, and after spring skiing and snowboarding at Vail, Colorado. I was a skier, but in my mid-60s I (and my wife) had taken up snowboarding to reduce the risk of an unrepairable injury to my artificial knee.

On May 13, 1999, the thallium scan at the Cooper Clinic seemed uneventful, but when I went back a few hours later to get the results, the doctor had a very concerned look on his face. His first words were, "I am not pleased with your results. You have major blockage in your heart, and if you lived in Dallas I would put you in a hospital right away." He knew, however, that I would insist on going home. The doctor gave me a pill immediately and three more to take with me. His parting words were, "Don't walk fast, don't lift anything, and get to a cardiologist right away." Waves of anxiety flushed through me, but after a couple of hours I slowly calmed down. Physically I felt great, so it was difficult for me to truly comprehend the severity of my heart condition.

While waiting on a plane at the Dallas/Ft. Worth airport I made an urgent call to a close friend with strong medical contacts in St. Joseph. The next morning I was in the good hands of Dr. Rowe in the cardiac unit at the Heartland Regional Medical Center. He found the blockage, performed an angioplasty to open the artery, and then deftly inserted a stent (small mesh cylinder) to keep it open. Only forty-five days before this procedure, my wife and I had been at Vail enjoying spring snowboarding—at 10,000 feet! I had no shortness of breath, no chest pain, not a hint of heart disease. It turns out that I am an asymptomatic type. My doctor at the Cooper Clinic told me, "Your years of aggressive exercise-walking built up a large collateral system around the blockage, which permitted your heart to get the necessary blood flow." Walking saved me from the "widow maker."

There aren't many 79-year-old guys writing exercise books. And I assume that most of my readers are younger than me. (It seems like *everyone* is.) I was your age once, but you haven't yet made it to mine. Getting to 79 wasn't exactly a smooth trip, and I hit a few physical potholes and speed bumps along the way. Since 1992, when the first edition of *Walking* was published, I have acquired *two* artificial knees, heart disease, and a stent in my heart, but I have also enjoyed some of the happiest and most memorable moments of my entire life. Whether you are 30, 40, or 50, if you start exercising now and adopt a healthy lifestyle, some of the best years of your life are yet to come. Believe me, it's true!

Chronologically, we all age at the same rate, but physically we do not. A sedentary 50-year-old may have physically aged more than an active 70-year-old. But by starting exercise and lifestyle changes now, you can turn your biological clock back and delay the aging process. Equally important, you will enhance your health, improve your quality of life, and most likely increase your longevity. As a regular exerciser, I can attest to significant benefits in all three areas, especially the last.

Even though I am a dedicated exercise-walker now, I want you to know that I failed to be a consistent exerciser at least six times over a twelve-year period. Let's be candid about exercise. A vigorous daily exercise routine for most men and women is unpleasant to contemplate, difficult to implement, and even harder to sustain. Don't be disappointed, and above all, don't be discouraged if you fail several times before exercise-walking becomes an important part of your daily life. Just keep on trying. Someday it might be the difference between life or death. It was for me.

From my normal weight of 180 pounds I had ballooned up to 232 in my late forties. I was fat! After several more unsuccessful attempts at exercise, I was finally able to make exercise a permanent part of my life at age 52. The nation was on a jogging craze, so like everyone else, I became a jogger. My wife joined me. Neither of us liked the jarring aspects of jogging, but it was effective. We both lost weight, and physically we felt better than we had in years. Three years later, however, I ended up with a knee about the size and consistency of an overripe honeydew melon. My doctor said my jogging days were over, and I became an exercise-walker by default.

I was physically fit and had lost 30 pounds by jogging, but now I had to walk for exercise. It was a downer. I couldn't walk fast enough to get my heart rate up for an aerobic workout, and

I was losing my good level of fitness. Even worse, I needed to lose 22 more pounds, and my weight loss plateaued. I was obsessed with trying to learn how to walk fast when I happened to read an article about the only race-walker ever to win an Olympic medal for the United States, Larry Young, who won the 50K bronze medal in 1968 at Mexico City and again in 1972 at Munich. He lives in Columbia, Missouri, only three hours away.

I contacted Young in Columbia and went to see him. He graciously showed me the fairly simple technique necessary to accelerate my walking pace, which I will share with you in this book. It was then that I decided to see how high I could take my fitness level with this walking technique. I came home and practiced, practiced, practiced. After a couple of years, I could walk 6 miles in 60 minutes. That was my absolute peak. (I forgot to tell you that I am one of those type A guys.) To find out what level of fitness I had actually achieved with high-intensity exercise-walking, I went to the Cooper Clinic. Many top athletes come there to have their endurance and fitness tested on the treadmill. To test for cardiovascular fitness and endurance, the treadmill is gradually inclined as its speed is slowly increased and the participant walks to volitional exhaustion. The clinic has compiled a chart called "Definition of Fitness Categories" for both males and females. The chart is broken down by age: under 30, 30–39, 40–49, and so on, and the total time on the treadmill is graded from very poor to superior.

The morning of June 3, 1985, as I got ready for my fitness test and the fifteen electrical leads were being attached to my chest, the attending physician smiled when he said, "If you are able to stay on for more than twenty-seven and a half minutes, you will equal Dr. Cooper's personal best time. He runs three to four miles four or five days a week at a seven-minute-per-mile pace and is two years younger than you." Twenty-eight minutes and 32 seconds later I stepped off of the treadmill exhausted but convinced that exercise-walking can not only give you the fitness of a runner but also turn back your biological clock. On the fitness chart my time was 1 minute and 32 seconds *better* than the time needed for the superior fitness rating of a male *younger* than 30 years of age. I was 57.

If you are a baby boomer turning 50 and worried about getting old, exercise-walking is the way to help your biological clock slow the aging process. If you are fighting a weight problem—it seems like our whole nation is—exercise-walking must become an important part of your daily life or it is unlikely you will win the battle. Most people aren't aware that walking, something we do too little of, can have such universal benefits. Unfortunately, walking as a form of locomotion in our highly mechanized world has been reduced to a minor role in our lives. The abnormal reduction of this fundamental human physical activity has led to obesity and a wide range of health-related problems on a national scale. For the extremely sedentary, it has even led to a reduced life span. That's the downside. The upside is that much of that can be reversed with an exercise-walking regimen.

Even though walking is the number one exercise in the United States, it is still not given the status it deserves by many exercise professionals. It is generally considered just an "entry-level" exercise for the unfit. In a nation obsessed with youth, speed, glitz, and glamour, walking is grossly underrated. Two important walking studies in this book that I have been associated with, one at the Cooper Institute for Aerobics Research (formerly the Institute for Aerobics Research) in Dallas and the other at the United States Olympic Training Center in Colorado Springs, clearly demonstrate that walking can produce more comprehensive exercise results than any other exercise or exercise equipment. You will find that walking is, indeed, the complete exercise.

This new edition of *Walking* is written from the perspective of a 79-year-old guy with a biological clock ticking at about 45. I'll try to motivate you "youngsters" to join me and the millions of others who have already discovered that a happier, healthier life is just a walk away.

Contents

Introduction

One of my great pleasures as a practicing physician has been to run across those occasional patients who live life to the fullest. A common denominator for these go-getters is passion, the kind of passion that drives them to excel when others fail, the kind of passion that keeps them motivated even when life lays down challenges. Those who possess this passion not only wring the most out of life, but also inspire others to do the same. Casey Meyers is one such person.

From the time Casey first came to our clinic more than twenty years ago I could tell he was passionate about exercise. And while his dedication to exercise was ostensibly to preserve good health, I could sense that there was something more. His dedication to activity was as much the result of how it made him feel as to what it did for his body. Such knowledge can be gained only through experience, and Casey had a lot of that. A long-term exerciser, he knew how beneficial it was to his sense of well-being, and was therefore dedicated to keeping it a part of his life.

Like many aging athletes, Casey has had to deal with his share of afflictions. A diagnosis of arthritis in both knees eventually led to total knee replacements. Undaunted by the setbacks, Casey has continued to exercise regularly. Even a diagnosis of coronary artery disease hasn't stopped him. He has undergone treatment with a coronary artery stent, and has done quite well. It is important to note that during his cardiac catheterization procedure the doctor commented on how his years of exercise improved the collateral blood flow around the area of the blockage, perhaps saving his life. It looks like Casey's passion for exercise to improve the quality of his life also improved his longevity!

Casey's exercise of choice is walking. This practical and effective exercise is one I know quite well. As a runner and walker, I can attest to its benefits. Walking was also very effective for me in my recovery from a knee injury I received while skiing in Colorado. Having recovered from my own injury, I know firsthand how effective Casey's program can be.

In this book you will find tremendous information on how best to implement a walking program that is right for you. He bases his recommendations on scientific studies and reliable sources. His style of writing is motivational, and his personal story illustrates just how much can be accomplished with the right attitude.

Yes, Casey is one of those occasional persons who inspires others to adopt healthy habits. I'm confident that you, too, will be inspired by his story and resolve to improve your own daily routine. All it takes is a good pair of walking shoes and a little passion.

Walking

ONE

Do You Have a Healthy Lifestyle?

You may be wondering why a walking book is starting out talking about "lifestyle" instead of walking. As a 79-year-old with years of hindsight to draw from, I am certain that this chapter on lifestyle is the most important chapter in the book. If I can't thoroughly convince you that you don't have any other viable option than to start exercising consistently to preserve your health, maintain your quality of life, and (I hope) increase your longevity, then I have failed, and you have wasted your money on this book. Please read this chapter carefully.

The large conference room at Missouri Western State University was packed for an April 2005 breakfast meeting, provocatively titled "Our Lifestyles Are Killing Us." The speaker, Lowell Kruse, CEO of Heartland Regional Medical Center, delivered a slide presentation that included a number of charts, graphs, and grim statistics about the current status of our population's health at the regional, state, and national levels. It wasn't a pretty picture.

The three leading causes of death in the United States continue to be heart disease, cancer, and stroke, in that order. A chart compiled by the Centers for Disease Control (CDC) and Heartland Regional Medical Center, titled "1990 & 2004 Leading Actual Causes of Death in the U.S.—Human Behaviors," caught my eye (Figure 1.1). Tobacco use is still the number one cause of preventable death related to lifestyle, but, fortunately, the number of deaths has not increased from 1990 to 2004. Even so, cigarette smoking still accounts for about 400,000 needless deaths annually.

The alarming category in second place was "Poor Diet/ Inactivity/Obesity." It shows a significant increase from 1990 to 2004 and is only about 2 percent behind tobacco. If its rate of acceleration in the last ten years continues, it will surpass tobacco before this decade is out as the primary cause of preventable death in the United States. As a nation, we are literally sitting and eating ourselves to death. *Our self-indulgence and inactive lifestyle are a deadly duo* (Figure 1.2).

Our daily lives are dominated by numerous reasons *not* to exercise. For baby boomers and all those born later, especially children born in the last ten years, what constitutes "normal" daily physical activity is vastly different from those of us born much earlier. I was a child in the thirties and a teenager in the forties, during World War II. In the thirties, obese people were uncommon in the general population, especially young obese

FIGURE 1.1
1990 AND 2004 LEADING ACTUAL CAUSES OF DEATH IN THE UNITED STATES
"Human Behaviors"

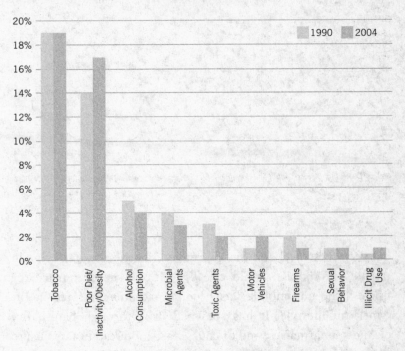

Source: Centers for Disease Control and Prevention and the Heartland Regional Medical Center.

people. Old films of World War II draftees in the early forties reveal lean groups of men. I was drafted in 1946, and there wasn't one fat soldier in my basic training company. It is quite the opposite today and has been so for several decades—especially the last twenty years.

Let's look at some of today's reasons our daily energy expenditure has been greatly reduced. In the early 1900s the marriage

FIGURE 1.2

CAUSES OF DEATH AND MAJOR ILLNESSES IN THE UNITED STATES

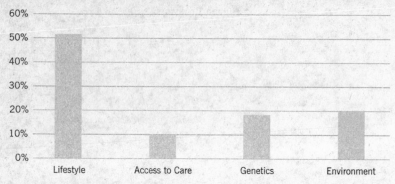

Source: Centers for Disease Control and Prevention, Presbyterian Healthcare Services, and the Department of Health and Human Services.

between the wheel and the internal combustion engine brought us the automobile. Amid cries of "It will never replace the horse," the automobile has become a dominant force in the American lifestyle. It has spawned drive-through banks, dry cleaners, pharmacies, and of course fast-food restaurants, just to name a few. We even have a drive-through Starbucks in my town. Other human energy savers include elevators, escalators, automatic washers and dryers, riding mowers, golf carts, power tools, automated assembly lines, moving walkways in airports, garage door openers, TV remote controls, and thermostats. With a furnace or stove, we used to carry in the coal and carry out the ashes, and in between we had to get up several times to stoke the fire. With today's heating and cooling systems and a thermostat, you can keep your house at an even temperature year round without moving a muscle. And these modern conveniences are just the tip of the iceberg.

In addition, we have actually *added* to our inactivity by spending countless hours watching television, playing video games, and surfing the Internet. The obesity problem for children is skyrocketing, but no wonder. Television has become a babysitter for the very young, who then graduate to video games. Sitting and more sitting. This raises an obvious question: with all of these wonderful modern conveniences, why would anyone in their right mind go out each day and spend their valuable time exercising and, heaven forbid, maybe even work up a sweat? The answer can be summed up in two words—*your health*.

From the very young to the very old, we have engineered ourselves into a deleterious state of inactivity. Unless you become convinced that a sedentary lifestyle puts your health and longevity at risk, it is unlikely that you will break the bonds of inactivity and be a consistent exerciser. Let me try to convince you.

The American Heart Association's (AHA) 2005 update "Heart Disease and Stroke Statistics" states, "Today, nearly seven of every 10 U.S. adults are overweight, and about three of every 10 are obese. And among children, overweight and obesity are rising at an alarming rate." The report continues, "Since 1991, the prevalence of obesity increased 75 percent, and obesity has increased among every ethnic group." According to the AHA, the estimated annual cost of obesity-related diseases in the United States is about $100 billion.

If I asked you to name the major risk factors for heart disease, you would probably say high cholesterol, high blood pressure, and cigarette smoking. You would be right, but there is one more that almost everyone misses. It is *physical inactivity,* also called *sedentary living*. In the mid-nineties the AHA added sedentary living to its list of major risk factors, giving it equal status with the most infamous cause of preventable death, cigarette smoking. If you are a nonsmoker but are sedentary, you are at a similarly high risk for heart disease. Sedentary living does its damage to the body slowly over an extended period of time just as cigarettes do. Most people in their 50s, 60s, and older tend to become more sedentary each passing year. And as the AHA report states, "While our level of activity declines, our rates of heart disease increase."

I would be remiss if I didn't emphasize that in terms of annual body count, the most destructive lifestyle of all is cigarette smoking. Year in and year out, it wins the death derby by a country mile. If you are a smoker, you can't walk enough miles or eat enough heart-healthy foods to undo the damage caused to your body by smoking. Dr. Tedd Mitchell of the Cooper Clinic says, "Nothing even comes close to smoking as the biggest cause of preventable death. It is in a class by itself." He added, "We know that smoking is a major contributor to premature death from heart disease, stroke, lung cancer, and emphysema, but cigarettes are also linked to many other diseases the public has not been warned about, such as pancreatic cancer." Many smokers have been able to quit, but unfortunately, many others have tried and failed.

Nicotine in cigarettes is a highly addictive drug that develops a tenacious hold on the brain's chemical receptors. Most cigarette smokers have great difficulty conquering this addiction when they try to quit. Cigarette companies have artfully characterized smokers as having the "smoking *habit*," because they don't want people to know that they are addicted to a pernicious drug. If you have tried unsuccessfully to quit smoking, keep trying. Nicotine addiction is far more difficult to overcome than breaking a "habit." In a strange twist of logic, some people (particularly women) continue to smoke because they believe it helps them stay slim. There is some truth to that, but they are trading a ham for a hot dog in that deadly deal. Life expectancy statistics reveal that cigarette smokers die eight to ten years sooner than nonsmokers. Smoking truly is a lifestyle that is killing us.

Obesity's role in our nation's escalating health care costs is now headline news. "Health Spending Soars for Obesity" was the headline for the lead story on the front page of the June 27, 2005, *USA Today.* The story revealed that private health insurance spending on illnesses related to obesity has increased more than tenfold since 1987. In April 2005 the prestigious Mayo Clinic issued a conference report titled "Action on Obesity: Report of a Mayo Clinic National Summit." In the report they listed diseases associated with being overweight or obese, which include coronary heart disease, congestive heart failure, hypertension (high blood pressure), type II diabetes, obstructive sleep apnea and other lung diseases, pulmonary hypertension, stroke, degenerative joint disease, many types of cancer, and gall bladder disease, plus a number of other diseases with long names that are unfamiliar to the average layman—including me. Many of these diseases are life-threatening and can lead to premature death.

Obesity is often determined by your body mass index (BMI). The BMI is a formula for adults, age 20 and over, by which you can determine if you are actually underweight, normal weight, overweight, or obese. Do you know which BMI category you are in? The formula by which you can compute your BMI with any calculator is as follows:

BMI = weight in pounds, divided by your height

in inches squared (height in inches × height in inches) × 703

For instance, if you weigh 220 pounds and you are 6 feet tall:

$$\frac{220}{(72 \times 72 = 5{,}184)} = 0.0424$$

$$0.0424 \times 703 = 29.8 \text{ BMI}$$

The following table (Figure 1.3) lists the BMI weight status for: (1) underweight, (2) normal, (3) overweight, and (4) obese.

FIGURE 1.3

BMI	Weight Status
Below 18.5	Underweight
18.5–24.9	Normal
25.0–29.9	Overweight
30.0 and above	Obese

The Centers for Disease Control website (www.cdc.gov/nccdphp/dnpa/bmi/index.htm) provides a full discussion of the BMI and also has a BMI calculator. Just plug in your height and weight and your BMI comes up with the click of a mouse. CDC cautions that two people can have the same BMI but a different percentage of body fat. A weight lifter with a large muscle mass and a low percentage of body fat, for instance, may have the same BMI as a person whose body fat percentage is much higher, because BMI is calculated using weight and height only. If you aren't lifting weights, your BMI may be telling you to lose weight.

The CDC cautions that it is very important to remember that the BMI is just one of many factors related to developing a chronic disease (such as heart disease, cancer, or diabetes). The CDC lists other factors besides BMI that also may be important to your risk of chronic disease: physical activity, diet, waist circumference, blood pressure, blood sugar level, cholesterol level, and family history of disease.

Another way to determine if you are overweight is to measure your waist at its narrowest point. It should be no larger than 40 inches for men and 35 inches for women. A Canadian study published in *Lancet* found that waist-to-hip ratio was also a way to determine if you are at risk for heart disease. Just measure your waist and hips with a tape measure and then divide your waist by your hips. Above-average risk for women is more than 0.85 and for men 0.9. High risk is above 0.95 for women and 1.0 for men.

The BMI and the other measurements are simply guidelines to alert you if you are at increased risk for developing a chronic disease. If your measurement numbers are higher than normal, the CDC recommends that you talk to your doctor to see if you should lose weight; they say, "Even a small weight loss (just 10% of your current weight) may help lower the risk of disease."

The April 2004 *AARP Bulletin* stated that the highest proportion of obese people (28 percent) was in the 50-to-64 age group, according to the CDC. The CDC's statistics also revealed that for Americans 65 and older the obesity figure drops to 19 percent—still high but an improvement. A CDC spokesperson said while there are many reasons why the older group has fewer obese people—some are thin because of chronic health conditions—"some obese people just don't survive into their 60s." This is a grim reminder that baby boomers who are obese need to develop a healthy lifestyle ASAP. Procrastination could be deadly.

If you are obese or are fighting an overweight problem, the weight-related diseases cited earlier by the Mayo Clinic are lurking in your future. I had a weight problem until I finally became a regular exerciser at the young age of 52. (Looking back more than a quarter century, 52 really does seem young.) If excess weight is your concern, you have my sympathy, because I know it is pure hell. Unfortunately, most of us tend to focus on our double chins and other aspects of our physical appearance instead of our *health,* which should be our primary concern. Without good health, everything else is irrelevant.

As I near the end of the longevity spectrum, I can tell you that status, image, money, power, and worldly possessions are meaningless if your health is gone. As the old saying goes, "You can't take it with you." When you get up into my age range it seems like everything either leaks or dries up, so you have to do whatever it takes to keep yourself healthy and functioning every day. Exercise is the key. Without exercise, I wouldn't be alive today to write this update. Someday, exercise may be a lifesaver for you.

A paragraph from my first book, *Aerobic Walking,* published in 1987, is more appropriate today than it was then. It comes from a study at Harvard's School of Public Health on the connection between exercise and fatness. The author stated, "In his hundreds of thousands of years of evolution man did not have any opportunity for sedentary life except very recently. An inactive life for man is as recent (and as 'abnormal') a development as caging is for an animal. In this light, it is not surprising that some of the usual adjustment mechanisms would prove inadequate." Simply stated, over thousands of years our physiological systems developed to function with considerably more physical activity than we are getting today.

The modern conveniences that we are surrounded with, plus an overabundance of food, rob us of our ability to get enough physical activity to maintain a healthy weight range. Generally speaking, if you are an overweight baby boomer, you should try to achieve the weight you were when you were fully grown and at your leanest and fittest. Old family photo albums will show that you were fully grown and probably at your prime weight in your late teens or early twenties. Heredity, however, plays a significant role in whether you are fat or thin in your late teens. In *Aerobic Walking* I quoted a doctor who said, "Fat parents usually have fat children who usually become fat parents." How to break that tragic cycle is the subject of much study and little agreement in the medical profession. Life is not always fair. You will probably have a relentless struggle between what heredity dealt you and your ability to maintain a healthy weight. Even with that burden, you may find that your best weight was still in your late teens and early twenties. To protect your health, the goal of returning to that general range is worth striving for.

Baby boomers who are fat now but had a fairly trim physique when they turned 21 can't as a general rule blame heredity. In most instances, the excess accumulation of fat that we often call middle-age spread is basically the result of caloric intake in excess of caloric expenditure. The surplus fat was deposited in the billions of fat cells we all have. These cells carry the normal reservoir of fat we need to fuel our bodies on a daily basis. When we inflate those cells with additional fat, we are simply taking on more fuel than we're burning.

The college textbook *Exercise Physiology: Energy, Nutrition, and Human Performance,* by William D. McArdle, Frank I. Katch, and Victor L. Katch, states that the average person has approximately 25 to 30 billion fat cells spread around over their entire body. When people gain weight and get fat they acquire additional fat cells. Someone who is extremely obese may have accumulated as many as 260 billion. Here's the kicker: even if you lose fat by the latest diet du jour, you don't lose any of the fat cells. That means those billions of fat cells will quickly fill up with fat again as soon as your caloric intake exceeds your caloric expenditure. How many times has that happened to you? It happened to me more times than I want to admit, but my weight hasn't fluctuated 5 pounds in the last twenty-three years, including holidays, vacations, and several cruises. What is the primary difference between then and now? Consistent exercise.

Exercise and increased physical activity are fundamental to preserving your health and achieving and maintaining a normal weight. Both are also necessary to break sedentary living's deadly grip. At the CDC a blue-ribbon panel of physicians and exercise physiologists met for the Workshop on Epidemiological and Public Health Aspects of Physical Activity and Exercise, which clarifies the difference between physical activity and exercise, which is confusing to many people. The CDC workshop defined *physical activity* as "any bodily movement produced by skeletal muscles that results in energy expenditure" and *exercise* as "planned, structured, and repetitive bodily movement done to improve or maintain one or more components of *physical fitness.*" *Physical fitness* is "a set of attributes that people have or achieve that relates to the ability to perform physical activity." Washing the windows or shoveling snow is physical activity. Walking 3 miles every day before or after work is structured exercise. Being able to do either without undue fatigue is a measure of physical fitness.

Physical fitness plays a significant role in extending our life expectancy. I remember vividly when Dr. Cooper told me,

"Moderate exercise, something as simple as walking 30 to 45 minutes a day at a brisk pace, will produce the moderate fitness level that is associated with a greatly reduced risk of death." A landmark study conducted by Dr. Steven Blair at the Cooper Institute for Aerobics Research, involving thousands of men and women over an eight-year period, was the first of this magnitude to prove a direct relationship between physical fitness and increased life expectancy (Figures 1.4 and 1.5). Equally important, the fitness level required to produce the most significant results is well within the range of the general population—that is, people like you and me.

Being fit enough to walk for four or five weekly workouts, each lasting about 30 minutes, slashed heart disease risk by 50 percent—even in men with high cholesterol—according to a study in *Circulation*, August 30, 2005. The study revealed that men who were physically fit were half as likely to die of heart disease as unfit men with similar cholesterol levels. Clearly, fitness at a moderate level contributes to our health and longevity. Getting at least 30 minutes of moderate-intensity exercise five or more days per week, or 20 minutes of vigorous exercise three or more times weekly, is recommended by the CDC to achieve a healthy lifestyle and increased fitness. Whether your preference is moderate or vigorous intensity, exercise-walking is your solution.

It is important to distinguish between different fitness levels when contemplating exercise. For health and longevity, you only need to walk at a brisk pace, as the charts in Figures 1.4 and 1.5 indicate. To increase life expectancy, a moderate fitness level should be the minimum goal of everyone. In my personal walking program, however, I am a high-intensity walker seeking a high level of aerobic fitness even at my advanced age. (My wife

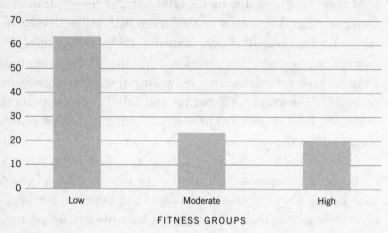

FIGURE 1.4
PHYSICAL FITNESS AND RISK OF ALL-CAUSE MORTALITY IN MEN
Age-adjusted death rate/10,000

FITNESS GROUPS

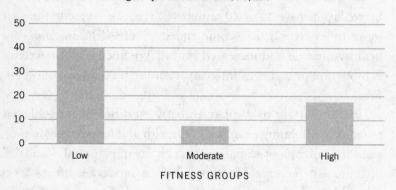

FIGURE 1.5
PHYSICAL FITNESS AND RISK OF ALL-CAUSE MORTALITY IN WOMEN
Age-adjusted death rate/10,000

FITNESS GROUPS

Source: S.N. Blair et al., "Physical fitness and all-cause mortality," JAMA 262 (17):293–2401, 1989.

claims that I am high-intensity in *everything*.) A high fitness level contributes to my physical capacity to snowboard, hunt, or perform any other activity without undue fatigue, but it does not necessarily make me healthier than someone who has a moderate fitness level. Both are good, and the purpose of this chapter is not to turn you into a jock but to convince you to break out of a sedentary lifestyle and to get you up and moving at any level that you will do *consistently*. Like taking vitamins, exercise is cumulative, and doing either sporadically does not contribute to your health.

There's a popular saying, "If it ain't broke, don't fix it." Although that may be sound advice for many things in life, when it comes to health, it may be deadly advice. By the time someone's health is "broke," it may be too late to fix it. The cumulative effects of an unhealthy lifestyle sometimes cannot be undone. The time to protect your health with exercise and proper nutrition is before it is broken. Dr. Cooper said it best: "It is easier to maintain good health through proper exercise, diet, and emotional balance than to regain it once it is lost."

People in their twenties, thirties, and even forties generally figure they still have plenty of time to lose weight and adopt a healthy lifestyle. They continue to eat, drink, and be merry. But even at these young ages, those who are sedentary and overweight are gambling with their health and their life. The many diseases, such as diabetes and heart disease, that are associated with excess weight and an inactive lifestyle are waiting in the wings to invade their bodies.

Baby boomers don't have *any* time to procrastinate on losing weight and adopting a healthy lifestyle. I was lucky when I finally became an exerciser at 52. I was sedentary, overweight, and unfit but had not yet paid a price in my health for it. Even though I became a dedicated exerciser, in the next twenty-five years I ended up with two artificial knees, heart disease, and a near brush with death. That's the bad news. The good news is, exercise and a healthy lifestyle also saved my life and gave me some of my happiest years ever. Over age 50, exercise and lifestyle become critical. The protective shield of youth is gone. Diseases that aren't even on your radar screen in your younger years are looming in your future. To protect yourself, the best health insurance you can acquire is a consistent exercise program and a healthy lifestyle. And both are free!

Having given you all of the medical reasons you should make a lifetime commitment to start exercising, let me give you the real reason regular exercisers continue to exercise year in and year out: *it makes them feel better physically and mentally.* In a conversation I had with Dr. Cooper on this subject he said, "Casey, even though we can prove that exercise can prolong life two or three years, I am not convinced that this will motivate people to exercise. Ninety-five percent of the people I know who exercise regularly do so because it makes them feel better, pure and simple." If I can make a lifetime exerciser out of you, it *may* help you to live longer, but I *guarantee* it will make you feel better physically and give you greater self-esteem and a more positive outlook on life.

I promise to put you on the road to a healthier, happier life with exercise-walking, but it will require some modest behavioral commitments. You won't need the discipline of a Carmelite nun, but you will have to get up off of your rusty, dusty rear end and start moving. Unlike other exercises you may have tried, exercise-walking will not bore you or injure you. With walking, I will show you how to take charge of your life mentally and physically in a way you never thought possible. You will exercise in a pleasing, natural way, but I caution you not to become impatient with walking; it works its magic gradually. Walking will take your unfit body and troubled mind and gently massage them into a state of readiness to battle life's problems or to enjoy more of life's pleasures.

I believe this is the most important chapter in the book because at this point you should make a lifetime commitment to yourself to protect your health. At 79, I know my time on planet Earth is getting short, but you "youngsters" have something on your side that all of the money in the world can't buy—*time*. Please don't waste it. The time to exercise and adopt a healthy lifestyle is *before* you have a serious health problem. Don't put off your walking program another day. Starting to exercise now while time is on your side is like heeding the old Chinese proverb "A wise man does not wait until he is thirsty to dig a well." I hope you will join me and start digging.

TWO

Walking: Its Origin, and Comparison to Running

We now have so many forms of mechanized transportation it is difficult to believe that for millions of years our only form of locomotion was walking. During my research for *Walking* in the early nineties, I read *"Evolution of Human Walking"* by anthropologist Dr. Owen Lovejoy, which appeared in *Scientific American* (November 1988). In his article, Dr. Lovejoy explored the origin of bipedal walking and its biomechanics. I traveled to Kent State University, where he teaches, to discuss this and another of his other anthropological accomplishments. Dr. Lovejoy helped to reconstruct and analyze the important 3-million-year-old female hominid skeleton that was discovered in northern Ethiopia in 1974. It was this skeleton that established our present knowledge of the antiquity of bipedal walking.

The anthropologists who made the discovery officially labeled the skeleton A.L. 288-1 but affectionately called her Lucy, a name taken from the Beatles song "Lucy in the Sky with Diamonds," which was popular in the expedition's camp at that time. Lucy was a small adult female, 3 feet 8 inches tall and weighing about 65 pounds. Lucy's skeleton reveals that she was as adept at upright walking as we are, and it proved conclusively that bipedality was fully in place three million years ago. Bipedal walking became the primary gait of locomotion for all of the species that followed Lucy and ultimately for us humans.

Dr. Lovejoy told me that our walking gait is about 98 percent identical with Lucy's. "The differences are just a few biomechanical subtleties. The most obvious morphological [structural] difference between Lucy and modern man appears to be the result of different degrees of encephalization [brain development]." Lucy had a head and brain about the size of a chimpanzee's. We humans, by contrast, developed a much bigger brain and have gotten smarter. Lucy could walk, but she couldn't talk. She did not have the ability to form words, since there was as yet no language. She had to forage for her food every day; there was no agriculture. The earliest recognizable stone tools are about two million years old, so Lucy was even a million years too early for the Stone Age. "It was only two million years from the first primitive stone tools to the industrial revolution about 150 years ago," Dr. Lovejoy pointed out to me. "In the last hundred thousand years, we went from Neanderthal to Cro-Magnon—modern man. Agriculture and domesticated animals came on the scene about ten thousand years ago; language, cultures, and religions appeared, and the wheel was invented. In terms of time from a geological reference, all of this occurred quicker than you can blink your eye."

In the last hundred-plus years we humans have invented new locomotion systems that have rendered our three-million-year-old walking gait nearly obsolete. Now the walking gait is viewed by most people in Western industrialized countries as the locomotion system of last resort. By riding more and walking less, we are shortchanging our physical activity requirements for a longer, healthier life.

Fortunately, over the past couple of decades, millions of people have rediscovered walking as a source of physical activity and regular exercise. Some doctors and exercise physiologists offer words of caution, however, and speculate on possible injury. Can it be possible that, after at least three million years of usage, the oldest form of locomotion is flawed? Or has walking been relegated to such a lesser role in our lives that we have forgotten that at one time it was the only way the human species and all of our extinct ancestors could move about?

An early example of injury concern was voiced at the CDC workshop I referred to in the previous chapter. In the section "The Risks of Exercise: A Public Health View of Injuries and Hazards," the three reporting physicians postulated: "Unknown are the injuries and hazards associated with walking and the rates at which they occur. We hypothesize that walkers share similar risks with runners." Fortunately, that hypothesis turned out to be wrong. Walkers do not share similar risks of injury with runners. Later in this chapter you will find out why.

They, like many others, view walking only as an "exercise" instead of our primary gait of locomotion. As you read this chapter think of walking and running as your gaits of locomotion to see how they differ biomechanically and why long-term walking is your best prospect for a lifetime exercise. Consider this: whether bipedal (two-legged) or quadrupedal (four-legged), there aren't any examples in the scientific literature of animals incurring injury—other than accidental—when functioning in their primary gait. Biological necessity is the sine qua non to the propagation of each species. The walking gait is fundamental to the survivability of all terrestrial animals. We humans are bio-mechanically designed to walk and walk and walk.

Walking works this way. If you want to go north, your back foot pushes against the ground in a southerly direction. A horse goes east when its alternating back hooves push against the ground in a westerly direction. "A quadruped has a greater amount of horizontal forward thrust than a biped; that's why we lost speed and agility when we became upright. In the quadrupedal posture, the center of mass lies well forward of the hind limbs. Our upright posture, in contrast, places our center of mass almost directly over the foot. We lose horizontal thrust and thus lose speed," Dr. Lovejoy explained. Center of mass is like a point on the body where, if you stuck a rod through it, the body would be evenly balanced in all directions, just as a wheel is around its axle.

To see what Dr. Lovejoy means by *center of mass,* observe the horse in Figure 2.1A, which has two circles on the front part of its body. The small black circle within the big circle around the chest, neck, head, and shoulders is its hypothetical center of mass. The overlapping circle, at the back, is around the large muscles and pelvis, commonly known as the hindquarters. That propulsion area is where the horse and other quadrupeds gener-ate their great forward horizontal thrust and speed.

Conversely, the circles on the human in Figure 2.1B are

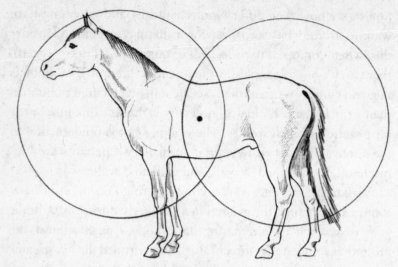

FIGURE 2.1A

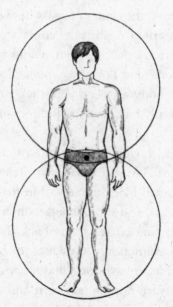

FIGURE 2.1B

stacked on top of one another. The big top circle is around the rib cage and upper body, generally called the torso or trunk. The small black circle within that is the hypothetical human center of mass. The overlapping bottom circle is around our propulsion system—the buttocks, pelvis, and legs. With this biomechanical arrangement, horizontal forward thrust is minimal. It is obvious that we aren't built for running speed like a quadruped.

You can easily demonstrate for yourself how we lack the forward thrust of a quadruped. Simply stand with your pelvis directly under your trunk, as in Figure 2.1B. With your legs together and straight at the knee, push against the ground with your forefoot. Notice that your ankles rotate as you push and that you don't go forward: you simply rise vertically, ending up on your toes like a ballet dancer.

The walking gait is a sequential lifting and falling of the body as our weight-bearing leg passes under us and becomes the trailing leg. The foot of that leg pushes against the ground, our trunk (or center of mass) is thrust up and forward, and then the trunk begins to fall. The lead leg swinging forward stops its fall as the heel is planted in front. This then becomes the weight-bearing leg as the body passes over it, and the process called the human walking gait repeats itself. That's how we walk. We all walk every day—we just don't do enough of it.

As we walk, certain muscles in the leg are contracting while others are relaxing. When the contracting muscles have performed their phase of the step, they relax while the other muscles start to contract and perform *their* phase. It is easy to visualize if you think of how the strings on a marionette work. Some strings pull the leg forward while others are relaxed. Four-legged animals move the same way. It is the combination of our unusual locomotion system and the development of our massive brain, however, that makes us unique in the animal kingdom. We have invented many ways to avoid walking, and we are too smart to do unnatural, boring physical exercise for long periods. Maybe that is why there are more couch potatoes than exercisers.

Dr. Lovejoy compared the human pelvis and its attached muscles with those of our closest living relative, the chimpanzee, to highlight the changes in musculoskeletal design. According to scientific analysis of deoxyribonucleic acid (DNA)—the carrier of heredity in our cells—there is a 99 percent genetic identity between humans and chimpanzees. There is great variation in our locomotion systems, however. Chimpanzees are basically quadrupedal, whereas we are totally bipedal.

In Figures 2.2A and 2.2B all the corresponding muscles for the lower bodies of the chimpanzee and human are identified with their proper anatomical names. Under each name in the human illustration (Figure 2.2B) I have added its familiar name if there is one. The need to stabilize an upright torso (as shown circled in Figure 2.1B) dictated the change of the gluteus maximus from a relatively minor muscle in the chimpanzee into the largest muscle in the human body, according to Dr. Lovejoy. The gluteus maximus is commonly referred to as the buttocks.

Some anatomists believed the gluteus maximus served as a major propulsive muscle in upright walking, but Dr. Lovejoy disagrees. He said, "When we walk or run, our upright trunk tends to flex forward at each foot strike, owing to momentum. The gluteus maximus has taken on the role of preventing our trunk from pitching forward. That's why it has hypertrophied [increased in size]. The gluteus maximus contribution to propulsion is limited."

When you walk you leverage yourself along the ground me-

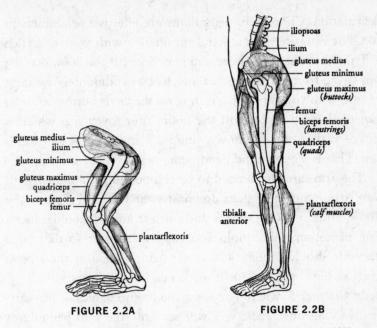

FIGURE 2.2A

FIGURE 2.2B

Redrawn from C. Owen Lovejoy, "Evolution of Human Walking," *Scientific American,* November 1988, pp. 118–125.

chanically and your legs function as pendulums. Dr. Lovejoy explained it this way: "The leg swing starts when the toe of the trailing limb leaves the ground. Like a pendulum at one end of its arc, gravity pulls it toward the other direction, and the iliopsoas gives the limb a tug forward to speed up the swing to the other end of its arc, where the hamstrings contract to decelerate and stop the swing. When the leg swing stops, you plant your heel, and the process reverses itself with the other leg." It worked the same way for Lucy three million years ago.

Generally, we don't think of the leg as a pendulum, but in fact our legs and arms are both pendulums. According to Dr. Lovejoy, they are *compound pendulums,* which calls for a bit of explanation. Compound pendulums are like two pendulums in one. For instance, if you stand on one leg with your other leg stiff and straight at the knee and your foot off the floor, that leg will swing from the hip socket, just like a pendulum. Now sit in a chair, with your upper leg resting on the chair bottom and the foot of that leg slightly off the floor. Your lower leg, which is hinged at the knee, will now swing back and forth like a pendulum. That is a compound pendulum.

The arms are also hinged to be compound pendulums. With your arm hanging straight down at your side and rigid at the elbow, you can swing it back and forth from the shoulder like a long pendulum. Now hold your upper arm out so that your elbow is shoulder high. The lower arm, hinged at the elbow, freely swings back and forth—two pendulums in one.

In Chapter 5, where you learn the biomechanics of the various walking intensities, you will see how the arm pendulums and leg pendulums interrelate. Not only do they counterbalance the normal walking gait, but, because they have the compound feature, they can be manipulated to help you walk at the speed of a jogger, to burn more calories, and develop a higher fitness level.

Figure 2.3 puts all the bones, tendons, and major muscles of the walking gait to work. If you take a full step, you can see the sequence of muscle activity—shaded areas—required to propel you forward. Figure 2.3A has the weight-bearing right leg angled behind the body, ready to push off with the toes as the calf muscle contracts and causes the ankle to rotate. At the same time, the quads on the front of the thigh contract to straighten the knee. The foot pushing against the ground propels the body forward. The right foot leaves the ground when the heel of the left foot is planted to stop the falling torso. Most people don't

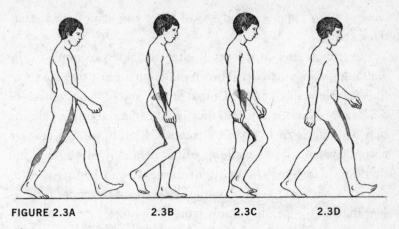

FIGURE 2.3A   2.3B   2.3C   2.3D

Redrawn from C. Owen Lovejoy, "Evolution of Human Walking," *Scientific American,* November 1988, pp. 118–125.

think of walking as a lifting and falling action. You can see, however, that as one leg is pushing from behind, you would fall forward on your face without the benefit of another leg swinging forward to stop your falling body.

Figure 2.3B has the left leg as weight-bearing. Gravity has caused the right leg to start to swing forward, and the iliopsoas muscle gives it a tug to speed its swing. In Figures 2.3B and 2.3C, the hamstrings contract to flex the leg slightly at the knee so that the foot will clear the ground as it swings under the body. This demonstrates the use of our leg's compound pendulum feature.

Figure 2.3D shows that near the end of the forward leg swing the quadriceps muscles contract again to straighten the knee before the heel is planted. The hamstrings contract to decelerate and ultimately stop the leg swing. The left leg is now angled behind the body and pushes off as the calf muscles contract. A complete step has been taken, and it has used *all* the major muscle groups in the lower body—just what you want for an effective exercise.

It seems entirely appropriate that our oldest example of the walking gait is a female. Women make up almost two-thirds of the exercise-walkers in the United States, and in the hundreds of clinics that I have conducted they tell me in a resounding chorus that walking is their favorite exercise. Rightly so. Women are natural walkers; their walking gait is definitely more fluid and rhythmic than men's. I know of numerous husbands who, to their chagrin, can't keep up with their wives. My gender may resent that, but it is indisputably true.

As my interview with Dr. Lovejoy was ending he said, "Casey, you can state in your book without any reservations that the bipedal human walking gait is at least three million years old. Not only was Lucy capable of walking upright; it had become her only choice."

When I got to my car, I sat there for a few minutes to let these words sink in. What a frightful predicament for Lucy! When she emerged from the primeval mists that shroud the beginning of life on earth, she was small, frail, and vulnerable. She had given up the ability to find food and safety in the arboreal world of her distant cousins. She was born a million years before even the most primitive stone tools. To move about for food, safety, and survival, Lucy relied mainly on her ability to walk and run. She could not run very fast, however, compared with the quadrupedal carnivorous predators with whom she shared her world.

RUNNING COMPARED TO WALKING

Many people who have a fear of flying generally defend their fear with the line "If God had meant humans to fly, He would have given us wings." To paraphrase this maxim as it applies to running, I believe that if God had meant humans to run for exercise, He would have given us the locomotion system of a horse. He surely would not have made us upright and two-legged.

This section will be informative for you because it will help you learn how your running gait functions in relation to your walking gait. I guarantee that you will take up walking with more confidence, pride, and determination when you find out that the only thing running can give you that walking doesn't is injury. You will become a true believer.

Walking has always been the recommended entry-level exercise for the obese and unfit or for older people like me. That's where everybody is supposed to start and then graduate to a more intense exercise such as jogging, running, cycling, or whatever. Having been a runner for three years before my right knee gave out, there was not one time that I truly enjoyed running as much as I do my daily walks. For me, running was always too jarring. I have to admit, however, that running helped me lose 25 pounds and develop an excellent fitness level.

The proponents of running recognize the injury problem, and the cover of an early nineties issue of *Runner's World* (February 1991) magazine reads, "Complete Injury Prevention Program at Last!" The opening paragraph of the story stated: "During the course of any year, you have a fifty-fifty chance of developing a running injury that will alter or stop your training. In other words, each year 50 percent of all runners, from recreational athletes to elite, sustain an injury that affects their running." The article was written by John W. Robertson, M.D., who said: "One of the best things any runner can do to prevent injury is to follow a regular stretching and strengthening program." This may help some, but probably not much.

As you learned earlier in this chapter, our center of mass is on top of our propulsion system. Unlike that of a quadruped, our musculoskeletal system takes a pounding from running, which predictably leads to injury—even in people who don't run very much.

A 1990 issue of *Fit News,* published by the American Running and Fitness Association, cited a study of three hundred male infantry trainees at Ft. Benning in Georgia. The men were divided into two companies. One company ran 60 miles during 12 weeks of training, while the other ran 130 miles. The injury rate was 33 percent in the low-mileage company and 42 percent in the 130-mile group. Ages were not given, but we can assume that a peacetime volunteer infantry trainee is in his teens or twenties.

A 33 percent injury rate for young men who only ran 60 miles in 12 weeks (5.0 miles per week) indicates that running as an exercise is seriously flawed. A 42 percent injury rate for the other group, who averaged 10.8 miles per week, is a pitiful statistic for a physical activity that is supposed to contribute to fitness, health, and well-being. Injury is the most frequent reason people give for dropping out of an exercise program. Once you understand how running works biomechanically as your secondary gait of locomotion, you will probably not use it as your primary exercise.

Because our center of mass is on top of the propulsion muscles, as shown in Figure 2.1B, with every running step we take, our entire body weight lands on a single foot that stops our falling body and then propels us upward and forward for the next step. Exercise physiologists calculate that we land with the force of three to four times our body weight; the figure 3.5 is generally accepted. Therefore a 200-pound man lands with the force of 700 pounds on each foot with each running step. This force is transmitted up the leg to the pelvis and lower back. Our musculoskeletal system does not have shock absorbers to handle such an impact. Something has to give—and over time it usually does. The history of runners with stress fractures, shin splints, knee, hip, and lower back injuries is well documented. You only have to look at how we are constructed compared with a quadruped to realize that we are not built for prolonged running.

The evolutionary role of running in all animals has been as a fight-or-flight survival gait to be used infrequently and in short spurts. Wild animals use running only as a survival gait. Dr. Lovejoy said he doesn't know of any animal that runs more than 3 minutes at a time in its natural environment. If you have watched any of the fine shows about African wildlife on public television or on cable, you have probably seen a lioness chasing a zebra. The lioness is running for her lunch, and the zebra is running for its life. The chase is brief. If the lioness doesn't bring down the zebra in a short run, she pulls up and looks for a slower one. The chase does not go on mile after mile, day after day; consequently, neither animal suffers injury from running.

Prolonged running not only injures humans, it also injures other animals who are better built for running. Of all the thoroughbred foals born each year, only about 50 percent survive training. Those that make it to the races often have brief careers. In a horse race, at the point of fatigue, generally in the stretch, when the horse naturally wants to slow down, the 120-pound jockey on its back starts whipping it. Many horses suffer injury when forced to run in a state of fatigue, just as human athletes lose coordination and tend to suffer more injuries when tired.

Stress fractures are a rarity among dogs except in racing

greyhounds. They are raced frequently for pari-mutuel wagering. Consequently, they suffer stress fractures that they would not experience in a natural setting. Stress fractures are common in human runners. In the "Questions from Readers, Answers from Experts" section of *Runner's World* (November 1986), a reader with a stress fracture asked for advice. The magazine's expert, a doctor, answered: "A runner gets a stress fracture when repetitive pounding and muscular action on the leg exceed the strength and reparative capacity of the bone. While an acute fracture is the result of a single traumatic event, a stress fracture happens because of repeated, less severe stresses over a period of time . . ."

Why don't horses suffer stress fractures when in a natural setting? *Equine Sportsmedicine News* (March 1988) explained how early horses moved about without human intervention: "The ancestor of today's highly regimented equine roamed the plains and forests freely, rarely staying in one spot long enough for the muscles to get stiff. He kept one ear to the wind so as to stay ahead of his predators, through continuous movement or short bursts of trotting. Running at top speed from a standstill was not part of his usual activity." And we call them dumb animals?

If running carries the excess baggage of injury, how did it achieve such wide acceptance as an exercise for humans? Running for exercise was given a big boost about thirty years ago, when Jim Fixx's *The Complete Book of Running* was published. Fixx's book was extremely well-written and inspirational to the point that if you didn't like running you tended to question your normality. Jim Fixx took a sport and made it appealing as a mass exercise. Until his book, most people viewed running as a spectator sport at high school, college, and Olympic track and field events. Yes, there were some exercise runners before Fixx, but as a percentage of the population they were few. Athletes who run in track events frequently suffer injuries, but it is considered part of the sport. Injury is accepted in every sport as part of the risk of the participant. Running at track and field events is a great spectator sport but as an exercise for the general population, running's role should be redefined.

Walking and running are our two natural gaits of locomotion. It is apparent, however, that we are misusing the running gait when we employ it for prolonged periods of exercise. *Misuse* is a different word from the one exercise physiologists and proponents of running use. They say most running injuries result from *overuse*. It will be easy, however, for you to understand why *misuse* is more appropriate than *overuse* for running injuries if you compare our biomechanical locomotion system with the mechanical locomotion system of a pickup truck. If a businessman or farmer bought a half-ton pickup truck and continually overloaded it with three to five tons, he would experience broken springs, bent axles, and a variety of other mechanical failures. The truck has certain performance limitations engineered into it. Similarly, our locomotion system is biomechanically engineered for the performance of unlimited walking but limited running. The breakdown of the truck is predictable; so is injury to an exercise runner. The problem of injuries from prolonged running is clearly *misuse,* not overuse.

Up until now, most of the information about exercise running has trickled down from its sports application, as a track and field event. Anyone who ran a 10K race (6.2 miles) or a marathon (26 miles, 385 yards) had to be aerobically fit and obviously used a lot of energy. Thus it followed that if all of us ran up and down the road for exercise, we would get fit and use a lot of energy. This is undeniably true, but zoological research on animals' gaits of locomotion—including ours—conclusively proves that running doesn't use as much energy as we once thought. If this is the case, then the primary reason that people jog and run for exercise is greatly reduced in importance. It was the research and considerate help I received from two zoologists—one in England and one at Harvard—that shed new light on the major differences between walking and running.

As explained earlier in this chapter, walking is the lifting and falling of our body as the trailing foot pushes off against the ground and the lead leg swings forward and becomes the support and weight-bearing limb. As compound pendulums, the legs have a natural arc-and-swing frequency; hence, walking is mechanical. When you break into a run, however, you shift (literally) from mechanical pendulum action to the elastic action of muscles and tendons.

The two critical phases that distinguish walking from running are shown in Figure 2.4. The walker (A) is in the *double-stance phase,* the brief moment when the front heel is planted and before the back foot leaves the ground. The *flight phase* of a runner (B) is just the opposite. Instead of both feet being on the ground before the trailing limb starts forward, both feet are off the ground.

Simply stated, a walker has at least one foot on the ground at all times, and there is a brief period when both feet are in contact with the ground. Conversely, a runner has a phase in which both feet are off the ground simultaneously and never has more than one foot in contact with the ground at any time. Whether you are going slow or fast, or whether it is called a jog or a run, once both feet leave the ground, you have shifted to your running gait and are using elastic energy in much the way that a bouncing ball does.

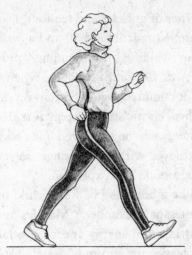

FIGURE 2.4A

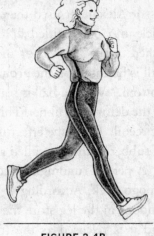

FIGURE 2.4B

You have shifted gaits many times, but you probably didn't realize exactly why. I am sure there have been occasions when you were late for an appointment and were walking at a pretty fast pace, then reached a point at which it was much easier to run slowly than to walk faster. That's when you shifted from the mechanical walk to the elastic run. Once you shift to a run, you are *using less energy (burning fewer calories) and less oxygen than if you had increased your speed by walking.* Please read this again and again and again. Most people don't believe it.

For over two decades R. McNeill Alexander, a professor of zoology at the University of Leeds in England, has been concerned with applying the principles of engineering mechanics to the study of animal and human locomotion systems. He is the author of a number of internationally published books, including *Animal Mechanics.* While researching *Walking* I contacted Professor Alexander, who sent me some of his research. It explains how our two gaits differ and function biomechanically.

To explain the elastic properties of muscles and tendons, Professor Alexander used the example of a rubber ball and a pogo stick in a paper titled "Human Walking and Running," published in the *Journal of Biological Education* (1984). When a ball is bounced on the ground, it compresses and flattens on the bottom. "When a ball is squashed, elastic strain energy is stored in the deformed rubber. This energy can be recovered in an elastic recoil. The same effect is achieved with steel springs instead of rubber in the toy called a pogo stick," he explained.

A person running is much like a bouncing ball or a child on a pogo stick. According to Professor Alexander, "Muscles and tendons in the leg store the elastic strain energy at each footfall and it is released as the foot leaves the ground." The elastic strain energy of running significantly reduces our energy requirements. He wrote, "This is how metabolic energy requirements are reduced to less than half of what would otherwise be needed." Running is our most efficient gait, and for good reason: in a fight-or-flight situation, if you are running for your life, you need all the help you can get.

All the solid materials in the leg have some elastic properties and must to some extent act as energy stores. However, Professor Alexander pointed out: "The skeleton is too stiff to be deformed much by the forces that act in running, so it cannot store much elastic strain energy. . . . The muscles and their tendons seem likely to be much more important. . . . It is probable that in running most of the elastic strain energy is stored in the tendons."

The suggestion that tendons serve as springs may seem surprising, but Professor Alexander explained it this way: "[The] tendon can do so because, although it cannot be stretched much, it is very strong and can store a great deal of elastic-strain energy." As an example, "experiments in which sheep tendons were stretched in imitation of running . . . showed that 93 percent of the work done stretching them could be recovered in an elastic recoil." As a comparison, "this is about as good as the best rubbers." Thus, exercise runners bounce along in nature's most efficient gait using elastic strain energy.

Here is an excellent description of how elastic energy is used in running: "During the early part of the stance phase, the muscles, ligaments, and tendons absorb concussion by stretching. As they stretch, they store energy which is released at a later stage in the stance phase to aid in propulsion. Recovery of this 'rebound' energy from the tendon and ligament springs is an energy-saving mechanism." It is interesting that this is quoted not from *Runner's World* but from an issue of *Equine Sportsmedicine News*. The muscles and tendons in a running horse function exactly like those in a human.

Even though our running gait is energy-efficient, we are slowpokes as runners. For comparative running times, Professor Alexander said, "A good human sprinter will race 100 meters in about 10 seconds at a speed of 22 MPH. . . . Most horse and greyhound races, however, are won at speeds between 34 to 38 MPH." An interesting example of a human trying to capture the horizontal thrust of a quadruped is shown in Figure 2.5. The sprinter gets a strong horizontal push against the ground and the starting blocks, but in a couple of strides the body is upright again and the running disadvantages of human biped locomotion return.

The biomechanics of the walking gait can best be seen in animated Figure 2.6, which shows that the center of mass (the black dot) is at its lowest point when both feet are on the ground. As the trunk of the body passes over the weight-bearing

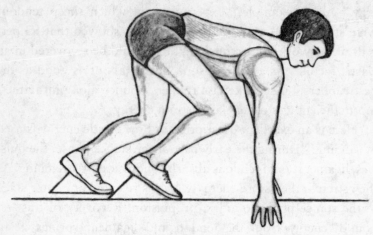

FIGURE 2.5

leg, the center of mass is at its highest point. It then begins to fall as the weight-bearing leg becomes the trailing leg. You can see that walking involves an alternate rising and falling of the body. It also involves alternate braking and accelerating; as the front foot stops the body from falling, the back foot pushes the body forward. This all works smoothly, and you are probably not conscious of the rising, falling, decelerating, accelerating activity that is involved with each step cycle.

It works very smoothly, that is, until you start to walk very fast. As you accelerate, you reach a point at which it is simply more convenient to switch from your mechanical gait, walking, to your elastic gait—running. Other animals do so for the same reason you do: it is easier and more energy-efficient for faster speed.

Researching my first book, *Aerobic Walking*, I acquired important zoological research on animals' gaits of locomotion and

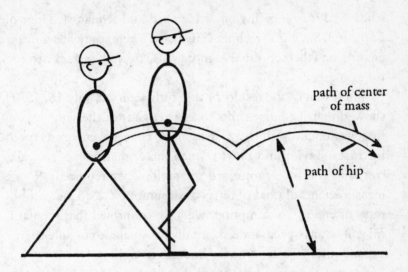

path of center
of mass

path of hip

FIGURE 2.6

why they change gaits from Professor C. Richard Taylor of the
Museum of Comparative Zoology at Harvard University. This
research convinced me that exercise physiologists are ignoring
the most important variable between walking and running—*gait
efficiency.*

I traveled to Harvard and talked to Professor Taylor about
his research. He and others have proven that human running
uses much less energy than might be expected. Once this point is
scientifically established, running for exercise becomes less desirable because of frequent injury, and walking moves up as the
best all-around exercise for the general population.

A horse in a field may be walking along and then start to trot.
After it trots a way, it may break into a full run. It went through
all three of its gaits, but how did it know exactly when to move
from one gait to the next? That question was answered in a

study by Professors Taylor of Harvard and Donald F. Hoyt of California State Polytechnic University. Their study has a direct bearing on whether it makes more sense to walk faster or to run for exercise.

Interestingly, the results of the study (*Nature*, July 16, 1981) showed that the horse shifts to a faster gait for the same reason that we humans shift to a faster gait: to conserve energy as speed increases. Taylor and Hoyt trained three small horses to walk, trot, and run on a motorized treadmill. They reported: "Using measurements of rates of oxygen consumption as an indicator of rates of energy consumption, we have confirmed that the natural gait at any speed, indeed, entails the smallest possible energy expenditure." This is true for humans as well.

Here is the part of the study that I believe is most important to you as an exerciser. Professors Taylor and Hoyt taught their horses to extend their gaits. By this I mean that when the horses would normally go from a walk to a trot, they taught them to walk faster. Further, when the horses would normally go from a trot to a run, they taught them to trot faster. Professor Taylor called this the "extended gait." Taylor and Hoyt wrote: "When the gaits were extended beyond their normal range of speeds, oxygen consumption was *higher* in the extended gait than in that which the animal would normally be using." This is very important. As an exerciser, if you want to use more oxygen to burn more calories, which calls for a higher heart rate to pump the oxygenated blood to the muscles, don't go from a walk to a run; instead, simply extend your walking gait and walk faster.

The ubiquitous automobile is the reason most people have drastically reduced their daily walking. Believe it or not, our gaits of locomotion have striking functional similarities to the mechanical gears in an automobile. One way to understand the biomechanics of gait efficiency is to compare it to an automobile's gear efficiency. For instance, if two five-speed cars are traveling side by side at 60 miles per hour and one is in third gear and the other in fifth gear, the one in third gear will burn more fuel and have a faster engine speed (more revolutions per minute) than the one in fifth gear. Thus, at 60 miles per hour, fifth gear is more efficient. Two automobiles with automatic transmissions produce the same results if one is locked in low instead of drive. Higher gears are used for higher speeds and fuel efficiency.

Gait efficiency in humans and other animals works the same way. If a walker and a jogger exercise side by side at a 12-minute-per-mile pace, the walker will burn more calories, use more oxygen, and have a higher heart rate than the jogger because the walking gait at that speed is very inefficient. Since the purpose of exercise is to use energy, the walker gets better exercise results (cardiovascular fitness and weight control) than the jogger, without the jarring impact or risk of injury that joggers and runners incur.

The application of the information developed in this study helps to establish walking as the most injury-free, sustainable, effective, and complete exercise. We all walk every day. We have been led to believe, however, that walking is of limited value when compared to running, especially for those who want an intensive aerobic exercise or who want to burn the most calories in the least amount of time.

Most exercise experts view a brisk 15-minute mile as the maximum pace for exercise-walkers. It is at about this pace or a little faster that people shift their walking gait into a run. That is the opposite of what you should do, and in Chapter 5 you will learn how to extend your walking gait to get the fitness of a runner without the risk of injury.

Before I leave this chapter I want all the readers who are biased toward running to know that I am not against running. Running is our other natural gait, and we can use both. Most exercise physiologists, however, compare walking and running simply as exercises without regard to the important biomechanical and gait efficiency differences between the two. The foregoing research by Professors Alexander and Taylor sheds new light on how we should view not only the effectiveness but also the long-term use of each gait as an exercise. In the short term, running can be very effective, but going back three million years to Lucy we are biomechanically designed to walk extensively and run infrequently.

THREE

The Specificity Principle and Walking Compared to Other Exercises

Have you ever heard of the specificity principle of exercise? Most people haven't, and neither did I until I learned about it while researching my first book, *Aerobic Walking*. This principle is invaluable in helping you choose a lifetime exercise, and the reference book I consulted, *Exercise Physiology* (J.R. Magel, et al.: *J. Appl. Physiol.* 38:151, 1975), explains it in detail. Here is an example you will readily understand. If you were a champion swimmer in top physical condition, you could not get out of the pool and automatically be a champion runner. Conversely, an Olympic runner can't jump in the pool and be an Olympic swimmer. The training and conditioning necessary to make the muscles fire and perform in one sport are not transferable to another sport. The training effect is sport-specific—thus, the specificity principle.

Exercise Physiology explains it this way: "Development of aerobic fitness for swimming, bicycling, or running is most effectively achieved when the exerciser trains the specific muscles involved in the desired performance." It concludes, "*Specific exercise elicits specific adaptations creating specific training effects*" (emphasis in original). To test this, the textbook cites a study of fifteen men who swam 60 minutes a day, three days a week, for ten weeks. The authors expected some aerobic transferability to running, but when they tested the men running on a treadmill, they found no effect.

If you are reasonably fit in one sport or exercise but tire quickly in another, *Exercise Physiology* states, "It is reasonable to advise that in training for specific aerobic activities like cycling, swimming, rowing, or running . . . little improvement is noted when aerobic capacity is measured by a dissimilar exercise. . . . Thus, one can appreciate how difficult it is to be in 'good shape' for diverse forms of exercise." When I read that last sentence, I wondered why we approach physical exercise any differently than we do mental exercise.

Everyone knows that if you are going to be a lawyer you study law, not basket weaving and applied pottery. If you are going to be an accountant, you study accounting, not first aid and canoeing. We all agree that we put the knowledge into our brain that we intend to take out and use. So why exercise from the neck down any differently than from the neck up?

Doesn't it follow that the exercise we put into our bodies should be something that has a residual value that we will use every day? *The only physical activity that we use every day is our walking gait.* From the time we crawl out of bed in the morning until we crawl back in at night, walking is our primary gait of locomotion. It has been since Lucy, and it will continue to be as long as the human biped exists.

In the course of the day, we substitute automobiles, riding mowers, farm tractors, or whatever mechanical device we need at the time for our walking gait. Even so, walking's role in our lives cannot be replaced entirely. For example, you walk from the house to your car, drive to work, park the car, and walk to your workplace. In the course of your workday, you walk from place to place. After work, you reverse the process. Everything we do is ultimately interspersed with walking. Our problem is that in our overmechanized world, we have reduced walking's role in our lives to such an extent that it leads to our physical detriment.

Based on the specificity principle, common sense dictates that *walking should be the foundation exercise for everyone.* Why spend 30 minutes a day on a rowing machine, for instance, knowing that when you get off it you won't be able to walk any better? How much rowing will you be doing during the rest of the day? Proponents of rowing will argue, and rightly so, that it will elevate your heart rate for an aerobic training effect and burn calories. As a walking proponent, I will tell you that by walking you can also get an aerobic workout, burn as many calories as a rower, and you enhance your walking gait so you can function better throughout the rest of your day—and for the rest of your life. Why exercise 30 minutes one way for half a loaf when you can get the whole loaf in the same 30 minutes?

THE OLD WALKER VERSUS THE YOUNG RUNNER

I had a personal experience with the specificity principle that I would like to share with you. One day in the spring of 1990 when I was on a national tour for a walking shoe company, I had a late afternoon to kill before an evening walking clinic. Across the boulevard from the Marriott Hotel in downtown Portland, Oregon, is a wide, paved path in a park that runs along the Willamette River for several miles. With the river on one side and the grassy park area on the other, it is a refreshing place to walk.

It was a gray afternoon with a little nip in the air, and there were a lot of runners and cyclists using the path this day as well as a few older walkers. I put on my sweats and nylon windbreaker and headed up along the river. I was cruising along at a fairly fast pace (about a 12-minute mile) when two young male runners came up beside me. They walked with me for about 20 yards, mimicking my bent-arm swing. We made eye contact, and I could see they were just clowning around. Finally, the one closest to me said, "Sorry, old man, this is too slow for us, we'll see you around," and they took off running. A few minutes later I saw them stopped up ahead, talking to a couple of female cyclists who were obviously friends.

As I approached, I could see they were talking about my walking. When I got to them I smiled and said, "I don't think you took off running because I was too slow. I think it was because you can't walk as fast as I can!" They took the bait. One of the guys said, "Aw, come on, walking is for old people. Anybody can do that." I took a fifty-dollar bill out of my windbreaker and said, "I'll bet you fifty dollars I can beat you walking down to the end of the path in front of the Marriott and back to here." By my calculation, that was a bit more than 2 miles. (As a word of caution, it is not wise to carry a lot of money when out walking.)

The one young guy said, "That's a safe bet for you because we don't have fifty dollars." I had suspected that when I made the challenge. I said, "Okay, I'll *give* you this fifty-dollar bill if you can beat me, and if you lose you don't have to give me anything." Now I had the girls on my side, and one said, "Come on, Steve, take him up on it. What have you got to lose? You can beat him." Steve, I found out later, was a 20-year-old college miler with a personal best time of 4 minutes 9 seconds for the mile. I'm glad I found that out *later* or I might not have waved that fifty-dollar bill at him. He just looked to me like a young runner who didn't have a clue about how the specificity principle works with walking.

After considerable cajoling from the girls, Steve decided to take my walking challenge. I said there was only one stipulation: his weight-bearing leg had to be straight when it passed under him so that he was not using bent knees in a flat-footed run. I showed him what I meant. Steve walked about twenty paces to try it and said, "No problem." We lined up to start. Steve's friend Brad stayed back at the finish line. We took off walking, and I could see that Steve's early strategy was to let me set the pace. My mile walk down to them had been just perfect for a warm-up. My walking muscles were ready, and my rhythm felt good.

I locked in at an 11-minute-mile pace for the first 6 minutes, and Steve stayed right with me. Young, fit legs are hard to tire, and at 62 my old legs were spotting him four decades. I kept checking my watch, and when we had walked 6 minutes I knew we were more than halfway through the first mile. By now my leg muscles were firing easily, my arm swing was loose, my rhythm was smooth, and my adrenaline was pumping. It was time to turn the heat up a little.

I increased my walking speed to about a 10-minute-mile pace for the rest of the first leg. We had gone about a quarter of a mile at that speed, and Steve was hanging right in there with me. A trickle of doubt started to seep into my mind.

A couple of minutes later, however, my confidence was restored. As we made the turn to head back, I glanced over at Steve. He had a bewildered, stricken look. Eyes speak volumes when fatigue shows up. I felt a new surge of adrenaline and confidence and decided it was time to see what this young fellow could do.

I have never race-walked competitively in my life. Out on my country walking course, I have timed myself at a 9-minute mile at least half a dozen times and once at 8 minutes 47 seconds. I knew if push came to shove I could do a 9-minute mile, and this was the time to do it. I kicked in the afterburners and took off. Steve was with me for about 40 yards, and then, as he told me later, his coordination was gone, his motor neurons wouldn't fire his leg muscles, his shin muscles were on fire, and he couldn't lift his feet fast enough for each step.

I was rolling now and widened the distance between us with every step. At this point, the only thing at issue was by how much I would beat him. When I reached Brad, Steve was about an eighth of a mile behind. Once he saw he was beat, he jogged in to give his legs a rest. When he caught up to me, Steve admitted that he had never experienced fatigue like that from running. The confusing thing to him was that when he sent a signal from his brain to his legs to move faster, nothing happened. His leg muscles had not been specifically trained in the walking gait to fire that fast over that distance, so when extreme fatigue set in they couldn't respond.

The old dogma that runners are more fit than aerobic walkers or race-walkers is as up-to-date as the flat earth doctrine. They are fit as runners only. Their specificity of running does not transfer to walking. It is a sure bet that a walker who can walk a 10-minute mile or faster will beat a good runner in a 2- or 3-mile walk if the runner hasn't cross-trained in walking.

I am 17 years older since I challenged the young runner, and now I don't believe you could throw me out of a tree as fast as I was walking that day. I am walking just as hard, but my muscles don't fire as fast, as my pace has slowed considerably. Nevertheless, the specificity principle becomes even more important as we age.

As you get older, it doesn't matter how fast you can walk, but instead if you can walk at all. Arthritis, strokes, and other infirmities that come with aging start to take their toll. For many my age, and even younger, walking becomes a daily challenge. Therefore, it is important to start as early as possible in life to exercise your walking muscles. The specificity principle clearly dictates that walking is the best exercise for you to achieve cardiovascular fitness and weight loss while maintaining your daily functional mobility as the years roll by.

LIFETIME EXERCISE CRITERIA

As you contemplate making exercise an essential part of your life and health management consider the essential items in the following list:

- *Exercise should be natural, not boring, and should be somewhat enjoyable.* Everything about exercise starts and stops with this. Nobody will stay with exercise if they dread it or if it is unnatural and mind-numbing. Exercise is a tough sell; telling you it's good for you just isn't enough. It has to make you feel good physically and mentally.

- *It should be injury-free.* It was injury that ended my exercise-running and forced me to find walking. Unfortunately, the majority of people who get injured doing exercise tend to abandon exercise altogether. Walking is natural and the most injury-free exercise of all. Don't give up on exercise until you have tried it.

- *Exercise should be accessible.* Sustaining an exercise program under optimal conditions is difficult for most people. If the chosen exercise is not readily available or takes an inordinate amount of time and effort to get to, it is easy to find reasons not to do it once the initial flush of exercise fever wears off. Your walking gait is with you 24/7, wherever you are. Use it.

- *It should be free.* The people who need exercise the most are at the lower socioeconomic levels. Getting them up and moving is an enormous challenge. If they had to *pay* for exercise, it would be an even greater challenge and most of them couldn't afford it. Even if you can afford to pay for exercise, why pay for something if you don't have to? Everyone likes bargains, and it doesn't cost anything to walk.

- *Exercise should involve the major muscle groups of the upper and lower body (preferably simultaneously) in a low-impact, rhythmic action that will permit the exerciser to achieve an aerobic training effect.* I have discussed these characteristics with a number of exercise physiologists and doctors, and they agree that they describe an ideal exercise. They also describe exercise-walking.

- *It should be possible to exercise at low, moderate, and high intensity levels in your chosen exercise.* This range of options in a single exercise permits the most sedentary and/or overweight person to start and continue in the same exercise up to a high level of fitness. I am not suggesting that you abandon any other exercise you like or are doing or that walking is the *only* exercise worth doing. If you are just starting an exercise program, however, and are uncertain about which exercise gives you the best all-around weight control and cardiovascular benefit for your time invested, then you don't have to look any further than exercise-walking—it is the complete exercise.

WALKING COMPARED WITH OTHER EXERCISES

Exercise is like a generic medicine, and all exercise has some benefit. Like prescription medicines, however, some exercises and exercise equipment are highly promoted and their results are often overstated. Some also have undesirable side effects. The following comparisons are to help you sort out fact from hype so you will not feel that something as simple as exercise-walking is less effective than some highly publicized exercises. You will also find that some of the other exercises work well when alternated with walking.

Cross-country Skiing

Cross-country skiing is a very good aerobic exercise because it uses the major muscles in the upper and lower body. People who live in the northern tier states, where they have heavy winter snows, can cross-country ski in the winter and switch to high-intensity walking when the snow is gone. The two sports are compatible. Cross-country skiing is a fun recreational exercise, and if you get a chance, try it. You will find as I did, however, that if you poke along slowly, your heart rate doesn't go up. Cross-country skiing is no different from any other aerobic exercise—it takes intensity to get a high fitness level.

Swimming

If you are a good swimmer and you like to swim, I won't try to change your mind. I would suggest, however, that you work in some walking to supplement your swimming. We are terrestrial animals, not amphibians, and anything you can do to condition your walking gait contributes to your ability to function on land. Remember the specificity principle: when you climb out of the pool, you will walk the rest of the day, and swimming conditioning does not transfer to walking or running.

In addition, swimming is not the aid to overweight people it was once thought to be. *Runner's World* magazine (October 1990) cited a study from the University of Missouri that compared the effects of exercise and diet on weight loss in four groups of regular but slightly overweight exercisers for a ten-week period. One group ran and dieted; another ran without dieting; a third group swam and dieted; and a fourth swam without dieting.

Randall Smith, clinical assistant professor of physical therapy and principal researcher of the study, said, "We noticed that swimmers are a lot hungrier than runners after workouts." Smith believes that the difference in appetite stems from the hypothalamus, the part of the brain that regulates temperature and appetite. Because water conducts heat away from the body more effectively than air, a swimmer's body temperature remains lower during a workout than a runner's. Smith believes an increased body temperature signals the hypothalamus to turn off the desire to eat.

Naturally, *Runner's World* was delighted to report on this study and reminded its readers, "If losing weight is your goal, stick with running." I will remind you that if losing weight without injury is your goal, stick to walking—especially aerobic walking.

Swimming has a couple of other drawbacks when compared with walking. The freestyle or front crawl, the most popular stroke, utilizes arm pull for as much as 80 percent of the forward motion. Your major muscle groups are in your legs, so not only are they not getting enough work, but they also aren't working against gravity, as they are in walking, because they are aided by the buoyancy of the water. Exercising against gravity is recommended for prevention of osteoporosis.

With all of its pluses and minuses, swimming provides excellent variety, especially when interspersed with exercise-walking. For those in the aging population with severe arthritis, swimming may be their only option. If so, go for it!

Outdoor Cycling

Outdoor cycling must be divided into two categories, exercise cycling and recreational cycling. The difference between the two involves speed. To achieve an aerobic fitness level from exercise cycling, according to Dr. Kenneth Cooper in his book *The Aerobics Program for Total Well-being* (Bantam, 1985), a cycling speed of slightly greater than 15 miles per hour is the optimal rate. He also says, "Generally speaking, speeds of less than 10 miles per hour are worth very little from an aerobic standpoint."

Cycling for significant caloric expenditure and aerobic fitness is difficult if you live in a city because of street intersections and the problems of traffic in general. In most cities there are very few places one can cycle nonstop at speeds greater than 15 miles per hour for 20 minutes or longer. For an aerobic workout, the heart rate should be maintained in the training range for about 20 minutes. Stopping, starting, and coasting cause the heart rate to fluctuate.

Consider also that the cyclist primarily uses the quads and very few other major muscle groups. If you've pedaled up a hill, you know that the fronts of your thighs seem to do all the work. When pedaling on the flat, the cyclist is sitting on his buttocks— the largest muscle group in the body. The upper body and its major muscle groups are hunched over the handlebars, totally inactive. Cycling injuries don't come cheap either. A fall at 15 miles per hour can mean broken bones.

Recreational cycling, by contrast, can be used to complement a basic exercise-walking program. It is fun and can be done at a leisurely safe speed as a light exercise. And don't forget to wear a helmet.

Racquet Sports

Tennis, racquetball, squash, and badminton are all great games. I was a squash addict until my knee gave out. Some level of fitness can be maintained if the players are competent enough to keep the ball or shuttlecock in play at an intense level. A hot squash game is a very good workout, as are the other racquet sports. But a game such as tennis doubles is not consistently active enough to keep the heart rate elevated. I view racquet sports as fun recreational activities. They are made even better by a high-intensity aerobic walking program. If you can walk 3 miles in 36 minutes or less, you will have more stamina and less leg fatigue, so you can enjoy your favorite racquet sport even more.

Aerobics and Aerobic Dancing

Aerobic routines come and go, as do the participants. The death knell for high-impact aerobics was sounded as far back as June 30, 1986, in a full-page story in *Time* magazine. It reported, "A recent survey of 1,200 students found that 43 percent had suffered injuries; among 58 teachers, the figure was an astonishing 76 percent." The injury rate should not be a surprise. As *Time* stated, "An aerobics dancer lands with a force equal to three times her weight." In the article, Peter Francis, a biomechanics researcher at San Diego State University, using slow-motion tapes, observed, "You see a rippling of the skin which is indicative of the shock wave traveling up the body." This high injury rate among participants and teachers spawned low-impact aerobics.

Exercise physiologist Dr. Michael O'Shea explained the difference between high-impact and low-impact aerobics in answer to a reader's question in the October 14, 1990, issue of *Parade* magazine. He said, "The traditional type of aerobic dance has been high-impact aerobics (HIA) which consists of jumping-type activities. . . . Over the past few years HIA has been associated with high injury rates. Shin splints, stress fractures, and tendonitis are common."

In an attempt to avoid injuries, aerobic dance instructors started teaching low-impact aerobics (LIA). Dr. O'Shea said, "LIA is described as maintaining one foot on the floor while performing large upper body movements with wide ranges of motion. . . . To increase intensity, the degree of difficulty of steps, cadence, and amount of work done by the arms versus the legs are varied."

It appears that low-impact aerobics is not injury-free either. According to Dr. O'Shea, it has been associated with hyperextension injuries of the shoulder. In addition, exaggerated movements place stress on the knees, ankles, and lower back. If you have tried high- and low-impact aerobics and didn't stay with it, don't blame yourself. Unnatural exercises, particularly those that induce injury, are not sustainable.

Step Aerobics

After high- and low-impact aerobics fell by the wayside, step aerobics was created. Fitness publications were quick to tell people what great physical fitness benefits they can get if they step up and down real fast on a bench that is between 6 and 12 inches high. There's more good news. If you swing hand weights around while you're stepping, your fitness supposedly doubles.

Frankly, I couldn't spend 15 seconds doing something as unnatural as step aerobics, but I know several women who go to a class a couple of times a week. They also walk the other days. Some exercisers like a class environment and exercising to music. If that works for you and it will keep you from being sedentary, by all means do it, but remember the specificity principle and do some walking also.

Exercise Equipment

I find many people are highly skeptical that something as basic as walking can be as effective for fitness as a piece of exercise equipment. There seems to be a pervasive belief that some unique physiological alchemy causes fitness to flow into the body from the machine. Don't believe it. All any exercise equipment does is provide a mechanical resistance, which you pay a healthy price for while the best resistance of all, gravity, is free. All kinds of devices designed for you to push, pull, and pedal are being marketed with slick ad campaigns touting them as fun and promising cardiovascular and aerobic benefits in a short amount of time. If you are not careful, you will part with several hundred to several thousand dollars before finding out that most of these devices aren't fun and the boredom of them turns your mind to mush. My foregoing comments do not mean weight-lifting and muscle-building equipment, however. I highly recommend them in conjunction with exercise-walking.

Exercise Cycles

An unsolicited brochure for a well-known and widely available exercise cycle came in my mail one day. The manufacturer claimed that this cycle burns more calories than other forms of exercise, but this statement is false. The company also claimed that you could get *all* the exercise you need on its cycle in just 12 minutes a day. That is also untrue.

The friendly price of this computerized exercise cycle was a whopping $1,675. You can buy a good exercise-walking shoe for about $70. If you took the $1,675 price of the stationary cycle and divided it by $70, you could buy twenty-four pairs of shoes. And if you were a pretty aggressive walker and wore out four pairs of shoes a year, you would be able to buy exercise-walking shoes for the next six years. On your next long walk, think how lucky you are, physically and financially, to be walking instead of pedaling your way to nowhere.

Stair Climbers

In a June 1990 article entitled "Stair Machines: The Truth About This Fitness Fad," *The Physician and Sportsmedicine* magazine stated, "There's nothing magical about the latest fitness craze." As the article pointed out, the obvious alternative to spending money on a stair climber is "just take the stairs."

Marketing of exercise machines such as stair climbers gives the impression that they can produce some magical fitness results and caloric expenditure in a very short time that exercise-walking cannot. I know quite a few walkers who spend some of their exercise time on stair climbers in the belief that they are getting concentrated results that would have required a longer time to achieve by exercise-walking. *The Physician and Sportsmedicine* quoted a director of sports sciences at a Denver health club as saying, "Many health club members seek exercises that expend a lot of energy in a short time."

The magazine also pointed out that fitness consumers want equipment with flashy computer screens that blink back physiological data (calorie burn, heart rate, and so on). The health club director said his clients will *wait* for a stair climber that has those features rather than use a noncomputerized device. But the accuracy of computerized stair machines is questioned by Bob Goldman, D.O., director of research at the High Technology Fitness Research Institute in Chicago, a nonprofit organization that tests exercise equipment. He points out, for example, that leaning on the armrests of a stair machine transfers less weight to the pedals and results in the computer's overestimation of calorie expenditure. Everybody I have ever seen using a stair climber was holding or leaning on the armrests; in fact, the advertising pictures show that position. More important, stair machines are programmed on the basis of the energy required to climb *actual stairs.*

The exercise equipment business is like Topsy—it just growed. Unfortunately, there isn't any government regulation to make sure these machines can deliver what they claim. Without regulations to guarantee the accuracy of computerized exercise results, the equipment manufacturers have free rein to overstate what their devices actually do without regard to the intensity and duration required to achieve those results. Meanwhile, people will continue to stand in line to climb to nowhere in order to have a computer give them caloric expenditure numbers that may be overstated.

The top criteria for a lifetime exercise are that it be natural, not boring, and reasonably enjoyable. Walking and running (or jogging) are the only natural exercises for humans. Walking meets all the criteria for a lifetime exercise. I believe that if the exercise professionals would recommend exercise-walking to everyone as their primary exercise, more people would exercise regularly.

Treadmills Are Best

If I lived in a city where traffic and air pollution forced me to exercise inside, or walking outside was not safe, or the weather was too hot, too cold, or too rainy much of the year, I would buy a treadmill. This is the only piece of exercise equipment that permits you to do the natural exercise of walking and complies with the specificity principle. Walking on a treadmill yields fitness that is 100 percent transferable to normal daily walking. No other exercise equipment can make that claim.

Here are six features that a treadmill should have:

- A minimum of 1.5 horsepower, preferably 2.0 horsepower or better. The heavy-duty motor should be quiet.
- Variable elevation, electronically controlled.
- Variable speed, up to 8 miles per hour.
- Ample, sturdy rollers and high-quality padded tread belt for a smooth walking surface. You should not feel individual rollers during foot contact with the belt.
- A walking deck at least 4 feet long to accommodate a long stride length.
- Easy-access controls: on-off switch, elevation button, and variable-speed button.

Those are the basics and all that you actually need. Some companies make a deluxe model with a computerized panel and all the bells and whistles and blinking lights. I suggest you just buy the basic, heavy-duty unit for considerably less money.

Here are tips on how to walk on a treadmill:

- Straddle the belt with each foot on the stationary outside deck and start at a strolling pace of 20 minutes per mile or less (3 miles per hour, if that is the calibration used).
- When the belt is moving smoothly, step on and walk at that pace until you establish the rhythm of your walk and feel totally relaxed and coordinated.
- Increase the belt speed gradually over several minutes, always making sure you have your posture, technique, and rhythm in sync.
- Increase your heart rate with walking speed rather than by elevating the treadmill. Try to walk fast with the treadmill flat or only elevated a few degrees to get your heart rate up. If you are unable to do that, then elevate the treadmill to

the level of a gradual hill and increase your heart rate by walking much slower.

- I believe it is better to reach your aerobic training range using a faster walking pace on a nearly flat surface in order to get your leg muscles to fire faster. This method gives you the residual ability to walk faster and with less effort in your normal daily walking. There may be days, however, when you don't want to work your legs that hard. By elevating the treadmill to a level where you can still maintain erect posture and rhythm, you can hit your aerobic training range walking at a slower pace. Experiment to find the elevation that feels right for you but try not to elevate the treadmill any more than necessary, so that you can always maintain correct posture.

- Do not hold the handrails. If you have to hold the handrails to keep your balance, you have the treadmill going too fast relative to your walking ability. You don't hold on to anything walking at your top pace down a road, so why should it be different on a treadmill? Let your arms swing freely.

- At a brisk pace, and particularly at an aerobic pace, walkers must have a good loose arm swing to counterbalance their faster leg swing. Just as important, a vigorous arm swing involves the major muscle groups in the upper body that would be inactive if you were holding the handrails. Never settle for half of the exercise when you can get it all in the same amount of time.

Do not be surprised if initially you can't walk as fast on pavement as you can on a treadmill. The moving belt aids your foot turnover from heel plant to toe-off. Even so, it does not take much pavement walking for you to catch up with your treadmill-walking proficiency. If you get your exercise at a fitness center, remember the specificity principle and do your workout on a treadmill.

YOGA

Yoga is something new for me in this update of *Walking,* and I strongly recommend that you give it a serious try. Yoga is an exercise of the mind and body that adds another dimension to an exercise-walking program. I was first introduced to yoga a few years ago at a Dr. Dean Ornish intensive weeklong heart seminar in Omaha, Nebraska. I was in my early 70s and frankly a bit skeptical, but with a diseased heart at my age, I would try sky-diving if it was supposed to be helpful.

I follow Dr. Ornish's heart diet (primarily vegetarian), but he also teaches that controlling stress is as important as diet and exercise in treating heart disease. We practiced a gentle beginner's yoga daily at the seminar and I stayed with it when I went home. That seems like quite a stretch for an old type A guy from the Show Me state, Missouri, but I have become a true believer in yoga and wish I had been exposed to it forty years ago. It might have helped prevent my heart disease.

Yoga, which originated in India centuries ago, has gained enormous popularity in this country. The word *yoga* comes from the Sanskrit word meaning "yoke"—that is, to bring together, to unite, to make whole. Dr. Ornish says, "It is a system that can help broaden a person's present experience of his or her own philosophy, religion and daily life." He adds, "The techniques are designed to increase our awareness of what is happening inside us—physically, emotionally, and spiritually.

Increasing our awareness extends our control over what is happening within. As a result, we can notice the effects of stress and make changes before they become full-blown illnesses such as heart disease."

In my research on yoga I encountered the writings of Dr. Jon Kabat-Zinn, the founder and director of the Stress Reduction Clinic at the University of Massachusetts Medical Center. In Dr. Kabat-Zinn's book *Full Catastrophe Living* he states, "Perhaps the most remarkable thing about yoga is how much energy you feel *after* you do it. You can be feeling exhausted, do some yoga, and feel completely rejuvenated in a short period of time." I subsequently bought his audio tapes that guide you through various yoga positions.

I use Dr. Kabat-Zinn's yoga tapes daily as an instructional guide to the yoga positions and, equally important, to pace myself slowly through the routine. Yoga should not be hurried; your mind and body should be in a relaxed, calm zone as you move from position to position. If you want to try his hatha yoga routine, his audio tapes are available at www.mindfulnesstapes.com. However, there are many other good yoga audio and video tapes on the market, and many YMCA and YWCAs have yoga classes. I suggest that you do not try to teach yourself yoga, but that you learn it from a reliable, qualified source.

In these stressful times, whether you have weight problems, marital difficulties, financial problems, or some other form of personal stress, the combination of exercise-walking and yoga will truly enhance your physical and mental well-being.

Finally, do not be intimidated by the pretzel-like yoga positions you may have seen in pictures. I have two artificial knees and cannot do many of the positions that require extreme knee bending. There are many other positions, however, that permit you to increase your strength, flexibility, and range of motion in the rest of your body. Progress comes slowly, and you are always encouraged to work within your personal limits. Do not set any goals; just let the yoga routine take you to your best physical and mental level.

FOUR

Walking Rx

Frequency, Duration, and Intensity

LEVELS OF WALKING INTENSITY

I believe the term *exercise-walking* is the most appropriate umbrella under which the various levels of walking intensity can be articulated. Two terms frequently used for walking are *fitness walking* and *health walking*. These are generic terms, but they are not quantifiable in relation to exercise intensity. *Fitness walking* has a nice ring to it, but we don't say fitness cycling, fitness swimming, or fitness running. People say that they cycle, swim, or run. It should be noted that *exercise* was specifically defined in the CDC Workshop as "planned, structured, and repetitive bodily movement." Thus, it follows that *exercise-walking* denotes a planned, structured, physical movement, as opposed to walking that is simply part of normal daily activities.

Walking has quantifiable intensity levels, and I will give them to you in minutes per mile. All too often walking pace is referred to in miles per hour, such as 3 or 4 miles per hour. Some people don't know how to convert miles per hour to minutes per mile; besides, runners never refer to their speed in miles per hour. A runner will say, "I run a 10-minute mile," not 6 miles per hour. It is much easier to compute your pace by knowing how many minutes it takes you to walk a mile.

Here are the measurable intensity levels for exercise-walking in terms of minutes per mile.

Strolling: Low Intensity

Stroll is a term familiar to everyone. It is defined in the dictionary as "to walk leisurely as inclination directs." Strolling constitutes most of our normal daily walking. It starts as slow as 30 minutes per mile and increases to about 18 minutes per mile at the top end of its range. Part of the definition, "as inclination directs," accurately describes how people arrive at their normal walking pace in the course of their daily activities.

Within the 30-to-18-minute-mile range, most walkers will find a comfortable, energy-efficient pace that suits their needs. The next time you are walking somewhere that doesn't require haste, check what kind of strolling groove you are in. The average person will comfortably stroll along at about 20 to 24 minutes per mile.

Strolling is the pace recommended for most people who are starting an exercise-walking program from a sedentary state. It is particularly recommended for the obese, cardiac rehabilitation patients, and the elderly. At the Cooper Wellness Program, where I conducted monthly walking clinics, we often had all three of these types in one class.

Obese people frequently have high blood pressure and are in a life-threatening condition. Happily, I have observed some remarkable long-term success stories about conquering obesity—stories that started with that first tentative strolling step on an exercise-walking program. Some obese participants found it a struggle merely to walk at the slow end of the strolling range, even for short distances.

Brisk Walking: Moderate Intensity

Brisk is also a term familiar to most people, and it is used frequently to designate an accelerated walking pace. In the dictionary it is defined as "quick and active; lively: a brisk walk." The brisk pace starts at about 17 minutes per mile at the slow end of the range and tops out at 14 minutes per mile. Most fit walkers can handle a 15-minute-mile pace comfortably.

Brisk walking is within the range of any healthy individual, but it is not the pace at which you should begin a walking program unless you are already reasonably fit. The walking booklet from the President's Council on Physical Fitness states, "Eventually, your goal should be to get to the place where you can comfortably walk 3 miles in 45 minutes. . . . We recommend that you walk as briskly as your condition permits."

Aerobic Walking: High Intensity

Aerobic walking is not a term familiar to most exercisers, but it ranges from about a 13.5-minute-mile pace at the low end up to a 10.0-minute-mile pace at the fast end. In this range, the two human gaits—walking and running—overlap. This fast walking pace is in the same range as a slow run or jog. Most fit walkers who learn aerobic walking generally level off at about 12 to 13 minutes per mile.

If you were formerly sedentary and progressed in fitness from a stroll to brisk walking, your heart rate may plateau slightly below your aerobic training range unless you increase your walking pace. If you want to increase your cardiovascular fitness level and burn more calories quicker for weight control, you will have to put more intensity into your walk to elevate your heart rate. The aerobic walking instructions in Chapter 6 will teach you how to achieve this intensity with exercise-walking so you don't have to switch to running or another aerobic type exercise.

Sometimes confusion over what to call fast exercise-walking occurs where you would least expect it. In the July 1990 issue of *The Physician and Sportsmedicine* magazine, Dr. Burton J. Lee III (physician to the first President Bush) revealed some of the president's exercise routines. Dr. Lee mentioned that at Camp David on weekends President Bush "sometimes conducts 'power walks.' " When the interviewer asked, "What are power walks?" Dr. Lee replied, "He just walks so darn fast that everybody disappears." That's hardly a usable definition of walking intensity, and I suspect that the president, who was primarily a jogger, was merely the best of a bunch of slow walkers. I would bet my quail dog—my most precious possession—that he couldn't have outwalked my wife, Carol.

An interesting sidelight: the second President Bush, a former runner, is now a mountain biker, according to a story in the August 22, 2005, issue of *Sports Illustrated*. They report he was an avid runner for decades, but had to stop pounding the pavement. As he said, "Like a lot of baby boomers, my knees gave out." Bush told the magazine that he gets "a great sense of ex-hilaration" descending a steep trail at 25 mph on a bicycle. He was only 59 when that was written. A few falls at that speed and his next exercise will probably be walking—and he will wonder why it took him so long to wise up.

I named my first book *Aerobic Walking* because it dealt with this type of walking intensity and the benefits derived from it. Terms such as *power walking, speed walking, pace walking*, and *health walking* are not quantifiable. What is physically challenging for one person may not be for another. Speed walking for some may only be brisk walking for others. By contrast, aerobic intensity is quantifiable. If you are walking and your heart rate is in your aerobic training range, then you are doing aerobic walking.

Race-Walking: Very High Intensity

Race-walking is a judged track-and-field event and has been part of the Olympic Summer Games since 1908. Race-walking is a competitive sport and not a daily exercise. In a later chapter, I cover the rules of race-walking and the technique necessary to become a competitive walker.

WALKING INTENSITY STUDY

The following walking study, which was inspired by the "extended gait" experiments of Professor Richard Taylor of Harvard, is my proudest contribution to the knowledge about exercise-walking. In the late eighties I was conducting walking clinics and consulting for the Naturalizer division of the Brown Shoe Company of St. Louis, and they provided a generous grant to fund this important study. It took place at Dr. Kenneth Cooper's Institute for Aerobics Research in Dallas, Texas, and convincingly demonstrated that increased walking intensity can produce the cardiovascular fitness level and caloric expenditure of a runner without the injury associated with running. The study was subsequently published in the December 18, 1991, issue of the *Journal of the American Medical Association.*

The study "Walking for Fitness—Walking for Health: How Much Is Enough?" conducted by Dr. John J. Duncan, isolated and tested the three intensity levels of exercise-walking: stroll (20 minutes per mile), brisk (15 minutes per mile), and aerobic (12 minutes per mile). The study was started in September 1989 and completed in the late summer of 1990. It involved 102 pre-menopausal, sedentary women with an age range of 20 to 40 who were randomly selected from the Dallas–Ft. Worth metroplex area. They all had to be nonsmokers, consume fewer than four alcoholic drinks a day, not be on a diet, and be free from cardiac, pulmonary, and/or musculoskeletal disease. They also were not to have exercised more than one day a week for the previous six months. It was important to start with a group of women who were sedentary but physically well enough to complete the required walking—especially the aerobic walking portion.

At the beginning of the study, I met with all of the walkers and gave them instruction on posture, stretching, and walking technique. Most of the participants were working women who wanted to break out of their sedentary rut and find an exercise they could do for a lifetime. They were eager to learn, and some of them even came at 6 a.m. to get their daily walks in before going to work. After thorough treadmill testing and baseline evaluation, the walkers started their supervised program. A control group was also tested and sent home to remain sedentary during the study.

The first sentence in the study stated: "Frequency, intensity, and duration provide the framework for developing an exercise prescription." In this study, frequency and duration were the same for all participants; only the walking intensity was varied. All the women walked five days a week. All groups started at 1.5 miles a day the first week, and their distances were progressively increased over the next 14 weeks until they all were walking 3.0 miles a day. This distance remained constant for the balance of the study.

The 12-minute-mile walkers were nicknamed the Green Berets because they were a tough bunch and liked the challenge of the high-intensity walk. I taught them the aerobic walking technique that you will read about in Chapter 6, and they picked it up easily. I want to emphasize that I did not teach them race-walking; they walked just like the brisk (15-minute-mile) walkers except they used the bent-arm swing technique. Walking distance, duration in total time and miles, and exercise heart rate were logged daily and were verified by a trained exercise physiologist, who supervised all sessions.

Perhaps the most interesting sidelight of the study occurred with the 20-minute-mile walkers. They started from their sedentary state fairly content with this slow pace, but in less than three months they were bored to tears. The women's average age was about 30, and they were finding that it was not only boring but unchallenging to walk this slowly day after day once they attained some degree of fitness. I got a call from Dr. Duncan, who said he was having a "walkers' revolt." Some of this 20-minute-mile group wanted to drop out because they didn't want to walk for three more months at this slow pace. We agreed to let the truly discontented ones increase their pace to 18 or 19 minutes per mile. Dr. Duncan held a meeting with the rebels and, with all the southern charm and persuasion he could muster, convinced them to continue at their slow pace.

One of the things he had to promise them, however, was that when the study was over, I would teach them how to do the aerobic walk. Part of their discontent was in watching the aerobic walkers zip by them day after day to complete their walk in 36 minutes instead of the hour it took them. To these working women, that extra 24 minutes a day was precious time.

There is an important message for all exercise-walkers in this sidelight. Even if you are sedentary and unfit when you start walking, in time your system will adapt to the slow, strolling pace of a 20-minute mile. You will find that a sustained slow pace is no longer challenging. All you have to do then is increase the pace of your walk enough to challenge your cardiovascular system again. This is where a heart rate monitor is very helpful. Don't make any abrupt, dramatic increase in intensity; simply pick up the pace gradually until you're exerting yourself during your walk and experience pleasant fatigue at the end.

WALKING INTENSITY MAKES A DIFFERENCE

The results of this scientifically controlled study can be used as a guide for anyone, including doctors who want to prescribe an exercise-walking program based on frequency, duration, and dose-related intensity. During the years that I gave walking clinics, better than half the people—and sometimes 75 percent of the women—were walking for weight loss or weight maintenance. Clearly, excess weight is a major concern in this underexercised, overfed nation. Since exercise is recommended extensively for caloric expenditure, let's review that part of the study first.

In regard to caloric expenditure, the study said: "If the primary purpose of the exercise prescription is for weight control and body composition improvements, intensity may be an important determinant." The old saying that walking a mile burns the same amount of calories whether you walk slow or fast is finally laid to rest. The study unequivocally stated: "Contrary to popular belief, we found that walking an identical distance at a lower intensity–longer duration does not provide the same kilo caloric [kilocalories are what we all refer to as calories] energy expenditure as walking at a higher intensity for a shorter duration."

To break this statement down into meaningful numbers, the study explained: "The gross rate of energy expenditure per 3-mile workout was 53 percent *greater* in the high intensity–short duration group (12 minute/mile) compared to the combination of low intensity–long duration group (20 minute/mile), and 26 percent greater when compared to the moderate intensity–moderate duration group (15 minute/mile). . . . Walking 3 miles per day at a 12 minute/mile pace, five days per week, would expend 30,680 more kilo calories per year than would the same walking program at a 20 minute/mile pace."

The additional 30,680 calories that an aerobic walker burns walking the 12-minute-mile pace represents almost 9 pounds of weight loss. (Note: 3,500 calories = 1 pound of body weight.) What's even more important is that those extra calories were burned while walking 2 hours less per week than the strollers. The 20-minute-mile walkers walked 5 hours a week to burn fewer calories than the aerobic walkers, who walked only 3 hours per week.

This was the first study measuring the 12-minute-mile level of walking intensity among women. A similar study of male college students, however, was reported in a President's Council on

Physical Fitness walking booklet. That study stated: "Walking's conditioning effects improve dramatically at speeds faster than 3 miles per hour (20-minute miles). At that rate, the college students burned an average of 66 calories per mile. When they increased their pace to 5 miles per hour (12-minute miles), they used up 124 calories per mile." This is only 8 calories shy of doubling the number of calories burned. Indeed, walking intensity dramatically affects energy expenditure.

WALKING TO THE AEROBIC FITNESS OF A RUNNER

Walking is continually excluded from lists of exercises vigorous enough to produce a top aerobic fitness level. The evidence is now conclusive that exercise-walking can be as effective as running or any other exercise for aerobic fitness when conducted at the proper intensity. Like caloric expenditure, aerobic fitness is directly related to the intensity level of the walker.

The cardiovascular system governs aerobic capacity, and heart rate reflects the amount of effort expended during exercise. *Aerobic capacity* refers to the maximum rate at which one's body can use oxygen. The aerobic walkers in our study demonstrated clearly that a maximum heart rate *can* be achieved by walking. The brisk walkers (15-minute mile) also attained an elevated heart rate, and Dr. Duncan observed, "For those who are interested in obtaining meaningful improvements in cardiorespiratory fitness, moderate to fast walking provides the necessary physiologic stimulus to accomplish this goal." For most, a brisk pace may be the pace they can sustain for a lifetime exercise.

I don't have a degree in exercise physiology; however, it was as obvious to me as an elephant in the pantry that if the two main objectives of exercise are to elevate the heart rate and to burn calories by using the major muscle groups in the body, the walking gait accomplishes both because it becomes highly inefficient and therefore requires more exertion the faster we walk. Why, then, are we continually advised by exercise experts to shift from walking to running to increase exercise intensity?

I believe the answer to that question is that most of those involved with exercise physiology focus on the difference of walking and running purely from the perspective of speed rather than gait efficiency. When the walking gait is elevated to a highly inefficient pace, as it was in the study, the exercise results are impressive (see Figure 4.1). The aerobic walkers (12-minute mile) exercised at an average of 86 percent (163 beats per minute) of their maximal heart rate capacity. The brisk walkers (15-minute mile) also did well. They trained at an average of 67 percent (126 beats per minute), while the strollers (20-minute mile) trained at 56 percent (106 beats per minute) of their maximal heart rate.

Once the walkers reached their assigned walking intensity levels at the 3-mile distance, their heart rates plateaued. The strollers (20-minute mile) could have strolled for another six months and their heart rates would have remained at about 106 beats per minute. As you begin a walking program, remember that the body adjusts to the demands placed on it. An exercise level that elevated your heart rate to your target zone last month may not provide enough intensity to do so this month. To increase your fitness from a lower level to a higher one with exercise-walking, you have to ask your heart to work a little harder by simply walking a little faster.

This was demonstrated by our brisk walkers (15-minute mile), who reached 67 percent (126 beats per minute) of their maximal heart rate during the last half of the study. That is a sig-

FIGURE 4.1
WALKING FOR FITNESS—WALKING FOR HEALTH:
HOW MUCH IS ENOUGH?

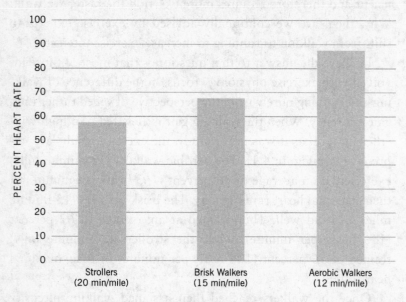

Source: Brown Shoe Co. Walking Study, Institute for Aerobics Research, Dallas, Texas.

nificant improvement from where they started, and it did not require any change in walking technique. Up until now, I have been comparing the fitness improvement and caloric expenditure differences between the aerobic walkers and the strollers, but it is time to give appropriate attention to the moderate-paced, brisk walkers. Their caloric expenditure of 269 was only 71 less than that of the aerobic walkers, and their heart rate indicated they were getting a good workout.

Brisk walking is a sustainable, doable pace for any healthy person who does not have a physical impairment in his or her walking gait. A good number of people in their 80s are capable of brisk walking. For most exercisers, the brisk pace may be the best because it is neither too fast nor too slow.

According to the study, the VO_2 max, which is a recognized measure of cardiovascular fitness, increased in a "dose response manner from the slower (+1.4 ml/kg/minute) to the moderate (+3.0 ml/kg/minute) and to the fastest (+5.0 ml/kg/minute)." The term *ml/kg/minute* is an abbreviation for "milliliter per kilogram per minute." Those words don't mean much to those of us who aren't exercise physiologists, but the numbers do. They indicate the level of VO_2 max improvement that these walking groups achieved from their original sedentary state and compared with the sedentary control group. The strollers (+1.4), brisk walkers (+3.0), and aerobic walkers (+5.0) all showed progressive improvement based on intensity. The study stated: "The VO_2 max differed significantly between the 12 minute/mile and the sedentary control group and the 15 minute/mile and control group, but contrasts between the 20 minute/mile and control group were not significantly different."

The slow stroll is the safe pace for everyone to begin a walking program, but, as the study indicated, if you never progress beyond it, you will not improve your cardiorespiratory capacity significantly. The reason is that the 20-minute-mile stroll is also the most energy-efficient pace within the human walking gait. It puts the least demand for oxygen on the cardiorespiratory system; consequently, it provides very little improvement of VO_2 max over the sedentary state. According to Professor Taylor's research on animal locomotion, animals usually select "an energetically optimal speed for each gait." It appears that a 20-minute-mile stroll is close to the energetically optimal speed for the human walking gait.

Establishing the VO_2 max improvement for the aerobic

walkers, one of the main reasons for conducting this study, was of great interest to me. I was curious about how their improvement (+5.0 ml/kg/min) would compare with that of people who run for exercise. Dr. Duncan said, "There have been numerous VO_2 max tests on runners, and the 5-milliliter improvement for our 12-minute-mile walkers would compare favorably to that of an average exercise runner." Figure 4.2, a chart constructed by Dr. Duncan, shows the percentage of cardiorespiratory improvement at the different walking intensity levels. Note that the aerobic walker's results equal those of a 9-to-10-minute-mile runner. The study results coincide with my own and my wife's treadmill fitness tests (superior) at the Cooper Clinic, which compares to fitness levels of exercise runners.

In addition to increased cardiorespiratory fitness, there was an increase in high-density lipoprotein (HDL—the good cholesterol) that amounted to a 12 to 18 percent reduction in the risk of coronary disease among all the walkers, regardless of walking intensity. The strollers did as well as the aerobic walkers, but it took them 2 hours longer each week to achieve the same results.

During the study, the three groups walked an accumulated total in excess of 20,000 miles. As the study stated, "Unlike most other modes of exercise, walking at higher intensities did not come at the expense of a greater risk of orthopedic injury." The study noted, "None of the women in the 12, 15, or 20 minute/mile groups sustained a walking related injury which necessitated consultation with a physician. . . . Thus, moderate-to-fast walking provides a safe and effective means for women to achieve significant gains in cardiorespiratory fitness." I've said it already in this book, and I said it at all my walking clinics: the only thing running will give you that walking won't is injury.

The proper prescription for exercise depends on the needs,

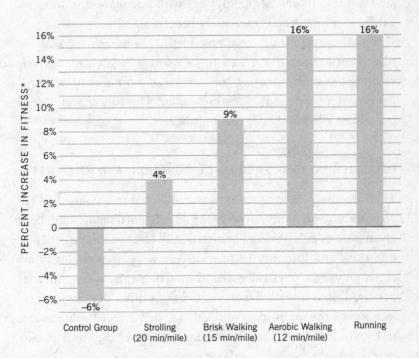

FIGURE 4.2

WALKING FOR FITNESS—WALKING FOR HEALTH:
HOW MUCH IS ENOUGH?

* As measured by maximum oxygen uptake.

Source: Brown Shoe Co. Walking Study, Institute for Aerobics Research, Dallas, Texas.

goals, and abilities of each participant. The walking study provided a sliding scale of intensity and amount of time necessary to increase cardiorespiratory fitness, cardiovascular health, or both. The study concluded: "For those interested in exercising for cardiorespiratory fitness or weight control, desired responses are achieved in a dose dependent gradient, with walking at higher intensities producing the greatest gains." There is a distinct difference between health and fitness. You can be highly fit and terribly unhealthy. For those only interested in cardiovascular health, walking frequently and with adequate duration, regardless of intensity, is extremely beneficial.

Finally, the study recommended: *"Emphasis should be placed on factors that result in permanent behavioral lifestyle changes while encouraging the pursuit of a lifetime of activity"* (emphasis in original). I promised Dr. Duncan that I would make sure everybody got this message.

ESTABLISHING YOUR FREQUENCY, DURATION, AND INTENSITY

The foregoing walking study was conducted in a controlled environment with daily supervision. Each participant had been given a thorough physical and treadmill test, and the frequency, duration, and intensity of the walkers were preset. Not much could go wrong physically with the participants, and no injuries occurred. If you walk five days a week, 3 miles per day, and select one of the intensity levels (20, 15, or 12 to 13 minutes per mile), you can expect results similar to those of the study participants, whether you are male or female.

Not everybody can walk five days a week. Others may be able to walk more. Is 3 miles the right distance for everybody? If not, how much is? The walkers in the study all started at 1.5 miles. Should everybody start at that distance? Once you have achieved a good fitness level, how much walking is necessary to maintain it? These questions should be answered and your initial fitness level established *before* you start exercise-walking.

This book will be read by people with a wide range of fitness levels. I won't be able to observe your tolerance for exercise, so I will assume that everyone is starting from sedentary. Many people get turned off by exercise when they rush into it from a sedentary state without regard for their physical tolerance. A number of things can happen—most of them bad. Above all, don't start exercising with the expectation that you will immediately experience some feeling of exhilaration and sense of well-being. Those feelings will come later.

When approaching any kind of exercise, it is always best to err on the conservative side. To establish your initial fitness level, approach it like putting your toe in the bathwater to check the temperature—very slowly and carefully. Finding out that you are capable of doing more is a pleasant surprise. Finding out that you did too much too soon is a pain in the buns—literally. The beauty of exercise-walking is that there is no reason for you ever to experience soreness or discomfort.

The most accurate way to establish a fitness level would be a treadmill stress test. If your doctor thinks you should have one, you should definitely follow his or her advice. However, for the average person (especially those under 35) who is starting an exercise-walking program, that is not necessary. All you need to do is take your first walk at a controlled, comfortable pace.

I recommend that you measure your walking fitness level in terms of miles instead of minutes. For instance, measure out a 1-, 2-, or 3-mile course in your neighborhood with your car odometer. Make a mental note of where the half-mile marks are. That way you will know approximately how far you walked the first time. Was it ½ mile, 1 mile, or longer? How far you went is more important than how long it took. Don't try for a fast pace. Whatever distance you covered becomes your fitness baseline. From that distance you will *slowly* add on the miles. Intensity comes much later.

In some big cities, where people walk in parks (like Central

Park in New York City) or in shopping malls, it is not easy to get exact distances. In that case, measure your first walk by how many minutes it took. If, for example, you walked 18 minutes, without any discomfort, your fitness baseline will soon increase from the 18-minute level. Whether you measure in minutes or miles, do not walk to the point of exhaustion. Always quit while you have a little energy left.

In establishing a fitness level, I favor measuring the walk by distance because, as you progress, your fitness level and pace will increase. The combination of distance and time is the best way to track your intensity level. An easy way to measure your progress is to check your time against a chosen distance. For instance, you may want to know how long it takes for you to walk 3 miles this month, then see if you can walk it even faster next month.

Frequency: How Often Should You Walk?

Is it better to walk 90 minutes one day a week or 30 minutes a day three days a week? In my walking clinics, the question of how many days a week to walk used to come up often. People who have the time and who thoroughly enjoy their walks should walk every day, or as many days as possible. As was established in the walking study—and in the 3 million years since Lucy— frequency does not cause injury.

Exercise-walking should become your foundation exercise for a lifetime. Approach it not on the basis of how little you can get by with but of how often and how much you can do. I can't emphasize strongly enough that if you are trying to lose weight you should walk seven days a week. Each minute and each mile that you walk you are burning calories and doing the best exercise possible for weight loss.

However, not everybody can walk every day, so the question is, how many days does it take to get some positive exercise results? In answer to the foregoing question, *Exercise Physiology* states, "Fewer than two days a week generally does not produce adequate changes in either anaerobic or aerobic capacity or body composition." We are not very concerned with anaerobic capacity, but we are with the other two. In a summary of six studies that investigated optimal exercise frequency for weight reduction, the textbook says, "It was observed that training 2 days a week did not change body weight, fat folds, or percent body fat. Training 3 and 4 days a week, however, had a significant effect. . . . Subjects who trained 4 days a week reduced their body weight and fat folds significantly more than the 3 days per week group." This is further evidence that walking seven days a week should be the goal for anyone in a serious weight loss program.

Other than for weight loss, the required frequency of exercise-walking depends on the level of fitness you desire and the intensity you are willing to put into it. For instance, if you intend to walk at less than the brisk 15-minute-mile pace, you probably should still walk five or six days a week. While this will give you only a low to moderate level of fitness, it will still benefit your overall health. Any exercise that contributes to your health is worthwhile.

Duration: How Long Should You Walk?

I have found that most people who become avid exercise-walkers end up averaging about 3 miles per walk. Time permitting, and especially on weekends, they tend to walk farther. My daily walk is usually 3 to 4 miles, whether I go slow, moderate, or fast. I am retired, so I have the time to walk 3 to 4 miles every day. This exercise time is as important a part of my daily routine as bathing or brushing my teeth. Unfortunately, there are millions of retired people in this country who don't walk at all. Walking even 1 mile would be a worthwhile contribution to their health.

Three miles per walk is a good exercise goal, and it is consistent with the recommendation of the President's Council on Physical Fitness. However, *Exercise Physiology* points out that "a threshold duration per workout has *not* been identified for optimal cardiovascular improvement" (emphasis in original). It concludes: "Such a threshold is probably dependent on many factors including the total work done, exercise intensity, training frequency, and initial fitness level." The variables of frequency, duration, and intensity are inextricably linked and can be manipulated to produce varying exercise results.

Intensity: How Fast Should You Walk to Attain and Maintain Fitness?

On the relationship of duration and intensity of exercise, *Exercise Physiology* states: "With high-intensity training, significant improvements occur with 10 to 15 minute exercise periods per workout. Conversely, a 45 minute continuous exercise period may be required to produce a training effect when exercise intensity is below the threshold heart rate." The textbook concludes: "*It appears that the lower intensity of exercise is offset by the increased duration of training*" (emphasis in original). Simply stated, if you are going to walk with less intensity, you should plan on walking for a longer duration.

Exercise intensity is essential in attaining fitness, especially aerobic fitness. Just as important, it is critical in *maintaining* fitness. In the question-and-answer part of my walking clinics, the following question often came up: "Will I have to walk every day for the rest of my life to stay fit?" The answer is that it takes persistence and the right combination of frequency, duration, and intensity to move a normal, healthy person from a sedentary state to an elevated level of aerobic fitness. Maintaining that level, however, can be accomplished with less frequency and duration than were needed to achieve it—as long as the intensity is maintained.

In a study cited in *Exercise Physiology*, healthy young adults using a combination of cycling and running 40 minutes a day for six days a week over a ten-week period achieved a 25 percent improvement in VO_2 max. They were then split into two groups, one of which reduced exercise frequency to four days a week and the other to two days a week. However, both groups exercised for an additional fifteen weeks at the same intensity and duration. In both groups the gains in aerobic capacity were maintained.

The same exercise model was used to study the effects of reduced training duration on the maintenance of aerobic fitness. Following the initial ten-week protocol of the other exercisers, these participants continued the same intensity and frequency of training for an additional fifteen weeks, but they reduced training duration from the original 40 minutes to 26 or 13 minutes per day. *Exercise Physiology* reports, "Despite this reduction in training duration by as much as two-thirds almost all of the VO_2 max and performance increases were maintained."

The only other variable to manipulate in exercise maintenance is the intensity of exercise. On this aspect, *Exercise Physiology* says: "When the intensity of training is reduced and the frequency and duration held constant even a one-third reduction in work rate causes the VO_2 max to *decline*. . . . *If exercise intensity is maintained, the frequency and duration of physical ac-*

tivity required to maintain a certain level of aerobic fitness is less than that required to improve it" (emphasis in original). The textbook concludes: "This strongly suggests that training intensity plays a principal role in maintaining the increase in aerobic power achieved through training." (The term *training* in this instance is used in place of *exercise*.)

The foregoing is extremely useful information for every exerciser, particularly for people who say they don't have time to exercise regularly and as a result don't exercise at all. I find that most people believe that once they start an exercise program they have to keep up the same regimen every day or they will lose fitness. This assumption discourages some people from making an exercise commitment. As the studies just cited show, this is not the case.

Exercise-walkers have great flexibility in maintaining their fitness levels by simply keeping up their intensity of exercise while reducing frequency or duration. The study cited in *Exercise Physiology* clearly shows that an exerciser can reduce frequency by as much as half and still maintain aerobic fitness. Getting an elevated aerobic fitness level still requires the initial commitment of three or four months. Thereafter, however, a lifetime of fitness can be maintained with more flexibility and in less time than most people realize.

How Quickly Is Fitness Lost?

Another question that came up frequently was, "If I have to quit exercising for a while for health or other reasons, how quickly do I lose my fitness?" When exercising stops, *Exercise Physiology* says, a significant decline in aerobic capacity occurs within two weeks. It further states: "After 12 weeks almost all of the training adaptations [i.e., improvements] return to pre-training levels." It doesn't take long to go from fit back to sedentary. The old saying "Use it or lose it" certainly applies to exercise.

The Aerobic Training Range

Adding intensity to an exercise regimen elevates the heart rate, and if enough intensity is added and maintained for 20 minutes or longer, an aerobic training effect is achieved. There are several ways to monitor the heart rate's response to increased exercise intensity, but the commonly used formula is the American College of Sports Medicine *Guidelines for Exercise Testing and Prescription:*

Predicted maximal heart rate (MHR) = 220 − age

The guidelines state: "Considerable variability (±15 beats min) is associated with this estimate of maximal heart rate."

Using this equation, an aerobic training range of 65 to 85 percent of maximal heart rate for a 40-year-old would be

$$220 - 40 = 180$$
$$.65 \times 180 = 117$$
$$.85 \times 180 = 153$$

Thus a 40-year-old's aerobic training range measured by heart rate would be 117 to 153. The guidelines caution: "The target heart rate range is only a *guideline* to follow in prescribing exercise" (emphasis in original). They add that judgment must be used about how an individual responds to exercise. If necessary, the intensity should be altered to provide comfort and

FIGURE 4.3
AEROBIC TRAINING RANGE (65 TO 85 PERCENT OF MAXIMUM HEART RATE)

AGE	20	25	30	35	40	45	50	55	60	65	70	75	80
65%	130	126	123	120	117	113	110	107	104	100	97	94	91
85%	170	166	161	157	153	149	144	140	136	132	128	123	119

safety while you are trying to achieve a training effect. Using this equation, Figure 4.3 lists the 65 to 85 percent training range for ages 20 through 80.

A word of caution: certain medicines, such as beta-blockers, alter the heart rate. Consult with your physician about what your exercising heart rate should be if you are on any type of prescription medication.

WALKING GUIDELINES

Using the frequency, duration, and intensity components of exercise, we can create some general exercise-walking guidelines in terms of how often, how far, and how fast. I emphasize that these are guidelines *only*. A walking program should ultimately match the fitness level, time constraints, and physical limitations of the individual walker and his or her personal exercise goals. One thing I am absolutely unwavering about, however: you should always achieve your frequency and duration goals before you attempt intensity.

How often: Four days a week minimum, up to seven days a week for those trying to lose weight. Unlike runners, walkers do not incur injury from frequency of exercise.

How far: Walk as far as possible without undue stress to establish your personal-fitness baseline. Gradually increase that distance to 3 miles, but do not increase it at a rate of more than ¼ mile every three or four days, or a total of ½ mile per week. Almost everyone except the extremely obese can handle this amount without soreness or unnecessary fatigue. I know many can do more, but it is better to err on the conservative side. If you are trying to lose weight, extend your walk as far beyond 3 miles as time permits.

How fast: For aerobic fitness, walk at an intensity that will put your heart rate into the 65 to 85 percent aerobic training range. In achieving your walking intensity, remember that *your heart rate is always more important than minutes per mile.* A high heart rate at a relatively slow pace means that you are not fit enough to go faster safely. As your fitness level rises, your heart rate will drop; then you can gradually increase your pace. For a moderate fitness level, use the brisk 15-minute-mile pace.

A good rule of thumb: Walk at least four days a week, and walk as far and as fast as it takes to achieve your personal exercise goals.

HEART RATE MONITOR

Next to a pair of good walking shoes, I believe the best piece of exercise equipment a walker can have is a heart rate monitor (HRM). Whether you walk slow or fast, knowing exactly how hard the most important muscle in your body is working is invaluable. This is particularly true for those who have heart disease and/or are older. I am in both camps.

My first exposure to an HRM was at the Cooper Wellness Program, where I was doing monthly walking clinics. The staff put them on all overweight participants and those who had some heart-related abnormality. The purpose was to make sure that the exerciser was not exercising too fast too soon. The most accurate HRM is a wireless unit with electrodes attached to a chest band that transmits your pulse signal to a receiver resembling an oversized digital wristwatch.

To check my heart rate I used to take my pulse for 15 seconds and multiply by 4 at the conclusion of a workout. This was okay but not very accurate. With a HRM you can monitor your heart during your walk to see if you should pick up the pace or maybe slow it down, depending on where your heart rate is and your level of fitness. Slow walkers, like the strollers in the walking study, will find that their heart rate will plateau once they achieve their frequency and duration objectives. If they simply increase their walking pace a modest amount, the HRM will show their heart responding by beating faster and working harder for better cardiovascular fitness.

Polar and Timex make two popular heart rate monitors, and both are good. I happen to use a Polar but wear a Timex wristwatch. You can buy either at most big sporting goods stores or on the Internet (Google "heart rate monitor"). I suggest that you buy just the basic unit—about $65 at 2005 prices. It lets you check your heart rate during your walk, and at the end it will compute your total time walked and your average heart rate. I walk 3 miles, so I can easily divide the minutes walked by three and get my minutes-per-mile average. It also has an alarm that can be set to go off when you reach a certain heart rate. This is particularly helpful for those walking for weight control—especially those who are obese—who want to safely walk at the upper end of their training range for maximum caloric expenditure.

I only wear my HRM about 50 percent of the time now because I have checked my heart rate during workouts for so many years that I can tell by my breathing and walking pace about where my heart rate is and if it is in my aerobic training range. For people who are just starting a walking program, however, especially those who have heart disease, are elderly, or are obese, an HRM is an accurate way to determine if they are exercising too fast too soon. When it comes to exercise, let your heart rate be your guide.

FIVE

Stretching, Posture, and Strolling

STRETCHING AND FLEXIBILITY

Over the years I have conducted numerous walking clinics for several thousand people, and I have found that less than 20 percent of exercise-walkers do any stretching of their walking muscles. Those who regularly stretch are usually the faster-paced walkers or race-walkers.

Flexibility is the ability of the joints to move through their full range of motion, thus allowing muscles to approach their maximum stretchability. Flexibility will vary from joint to joint and person to person. Don't be alarmed if you can't attain the same flexibility that your walking partner can. Simply work on getting the maximum flexibility possible for you. An exercise-walker uses all the major muscle groups in the lower body; stretching these muscles and making sure the joints they influence are flexible are important for a fluid, rhythmic walk.

The type of stretching you should do is called *static stretching*, which simply means that you stretch the muscle slowly to its greatest possible length and hold it for about 10 to 20 seconds. Then slowly release the tension on the muscle. Stretch until you feel a pulling sensation, with a slight bit of discomfort or a minor, dull ache. You should not feel pain, and above all you should not bounce or snap the muscle. Over time, stretching will produce a semipermanent lengthening of the muscle; if you stop stretching, the muscle will soon shorten again, especially if you are older. I can say amen to that.

There are many ways to stretch the same muscle or muscle group. I have chosen the exercises that I think are the easiest to do anywhere. A great many stretches require being on the ground or on the floor. I have eliminated those because if you are walking outdoors or in a shopping mall, you probably would not want to get down on the ground or the floor. It is best to warm up with the type of exercise you are going to do. Runners jog and walkers walk. Warm muscles are more elastic, and their stretching is more effective.

If you are just starting a stretching and flexibility program, repeat each stretching exercise three times and hold the stretch for a count of 10 seconds. As your flexibility increases, hold the stretch for a count of 20 to 30 seconds and do five repetitions. Remember to breathe normally. Like all exercises, stretching takes more effort and frequency to improve from zero to a desirable level than it does to maintain that level. You should perform the stretching exercises three to five days per week to *increase* flexibility, but you only need to do them two to three days per week to *maintain* flexibility. More than five days per week is not necessary.

I am going to show you three priority stretches that I guarantee will help you walk better. These stretches involve the muscles or muscle groups that contribute to the walking gait. Obviously, from an overall flexibility standpoint we should do more stretches, but this chapter is concerned only with getting your walking program started.

The muscle groups that contribute most to the walking gait are (1) hamstrings (back of the thighs), (2) calf muscles, and (3) quadriceps (front of the thighs). It is a close call whether the calf muscles are more important than the hamstrings. Some racewalking coaches will argue that they are. From a pure propulsion standpoint, that may be true, but I have found that most people (especially older people) need to work more on their shortened hamstrings than on their calf muscles, so we will start with them.

Hamstrings Stretch

As explained in Chapter 2, the main function of the hamstrings is to decelerate and stop the leg on the forward swing so the walker can plant his or her heel. The hamstrings are attached to both the back of the knee and the pelvis. They flex the knee at toe-off as the leg starts its forward swing, lifting the foot and permitting the toes to clear the ground as the foot passes under the body. Shortened hamstrings cause shortened stride lengths. If your hamstrings cannot reach their full extension at the end of the forward leg swing, the heel of your front foot will land at a shorter distance from your back foot than it normally would. You will have a short, choppy stride.

There are many ways to stretch the hamstrings, but the one in the illustration (see Figure 5.1) seems to be the simplest and most adaptable to various exercise situations. I like it because it doesn't require extensive bending of the back or getting on the floor. I have one of those backs that doesn't straighten up every time I bend over.

Stand with one foot on a chair, a park bench, or even the bumper of your car, with the toes of the elevated foot pointing straight up. Make sure both legs are straight and the knees locked. There is a tendency to bend the knee of the weight-bearing leg, but keep it straight at all times. Place your hands on your hips and *slowly* bend forward, trying to touch your nose to the knee of your raised leg. You will immediately feel the tension in the hamstring muscles in your raised leg. *Don't bounce*. After the count of 10, straighten up slowly and reverse legs.

Calf Muscles and Tendon Stretch

The calf muscles supply the main propulsion of the walking gait. They are no strangers to most people because at one time or another we have all had calf cramps. Sometimes getting the toes of a foot extended under the covers in bed at night can cause the calf to knot up and make you think a pit bull has you by the leg. It is worthwhile to see the calf muscles in an anatomical illustration (Figure 5.2).

The upper calf muscles are called the gastrocnemius; the lower calf muscles are the soleus. As a group, these muscles are called the triceps surae. The Achilles tendon hooks the calf muscles to the heel. As your weight-bearing foot passes under your body and becomes the trailing limb, your heel rises and your forefoot pushes against the ground toward toe-off. This motion

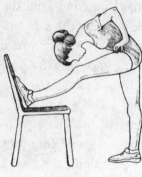

FIGURE 5.1

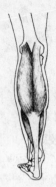

FIGURE 5.2

is accomplished by a short, powerful contraction of the calf muscles. You can readily see why having these muscles functioning at their maximum potential will contribute to your walking propulsion.

Upper Calf Muscle Stretch

Stand with your feet about 18 inches apart and 3 or 4 feet from a wall (or tree, if you are outside). As in Figure 5.3, lean forward with your back straight and place both hands on the tree. Slowly bring your hips forward while keeping your legs straight and your heels flat on the ground. There is a natural tendency for the heels to rise. Keep them down and you will feel the pull on the upper calf muscles in both legs. Hold this position for the count of 10 (for beginners), then ease back with your hips. Repeat a total of three times.

Lower Calf Muscle and Achilles Tendon Stretch

As in Figure 5.4, with your feet, hands, and body in the same position as in the previous stretch, slowly bend your knees as if you were going to squat, but be sure to keep your heels flat on the

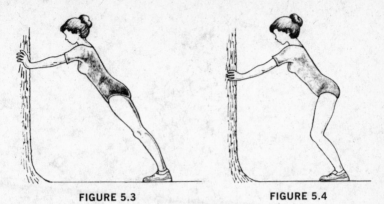

FIGURE 5.3   FIGURE 5.4

floor. You will feel the pull on the lower calf muscles and
Achilles tendons. Hold for the appropriate count, then slowly
rise. Alternate the lower stretch with the upper stretch for the
appropriate number of repetitions.

Quadriceps Stretch

The big muscle group on the front of the thighs is commonly
called the quads. They straighten the knee as your swing leg
comes forward just before you plant your heel. They are connected to the patellar tendon, which goes down over the kneecap
and attaches to the front of the upper part of the lower leg.

When you make your hamstrings flex your knee by pulling
the lower leg up, the quads are the muscles that pull on the front
of the lower leg to extend your knee and straighten the leg.
Quads get their biggest workout when you are walking up a hill
or up stairs. They lift your body as they straighten the knee.

Stand next to a wall or tree for balance. As in Figure 5.5, reach
back and slowly pull your non-weight-bearing foot up toward
your buttocks until you feel the tension or a minor, dull ache in

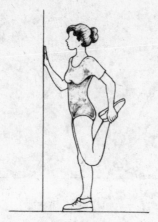

FIGURE 5.5

the front thigh muscles. Don't pull the foot up sharply. Hold for the appropriate count, then switch legs. You should ultimately be able to touch your heels to your buttocks. People with knee problems may not be able to get a full quad stretch, however. I used to be able to get a full stretch, but now with two artificial knees I can barely get a half stretch. If you have arthritis or other knee problems, do the best you can and take what you can get.

There is no question that if you do these three stretches you will get more out of your exercise walk and will function better in your normal daily walking. I can't emphasize strongly enough that the older you get, the more important stretching and flexibility become.

Hip and Trunk Flexion

There are two stretches that I recommend that you do each day *after* your walk. These stretches are not directly related to the propulsion of your walking gait, but they give you flexibility in an important area—the lower and middle back. Anyone who has had pain in the lower back knows the meaning of misery. Even a cough or a sneeze can make you think you are coming unhinged. These two stretches are easy and effective.

Hip Flexion

Lie on your back and grasp your knees (see Figure 5.6). Contract the abdominal muscles and pull your knees to your chest while pressing your lower back to the floor. If you have knee problems, pull from behind the knee at the lower end of your upper leg. Hold this position for the appropriate count, then relax a moment and repeat. Do this stretch several times a week.

Middle and Lower Back Stretch

Sit on a firm chair and spread your knees. As in Figure 5.7, slowly bend forward, with your arms outstretched and your hands together. Reach for the floor as far forward as possible with your hands and hold for the appropriate count. You will feel the pull in the lower and middle back. Do this stretch several times a week also. Those who have a potbelly will find they can't get very far down on this one. Keep trying anyhow! We'll work on that potbelly in a later chapter.

When to Stretch

According to every authority on stretching that I have researched, the proper procedure is:

1. Warm up.
2. Do your stretching routine.

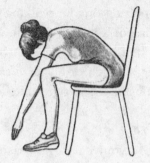

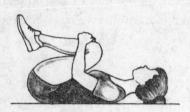

FIGURE 5.6   FIGURE 5.7

3. Engage in your exercise or sport.
4. Stretch again when you are finished and the muscles are still warm.

Now let's talk about the real world. Eighty percent of the population doesn't exercise at all. Of those who are currently exercise-walking, less than 20 percent are doing any stretching.

I have found that walking a few minutes to warm up, stopping to stretch, and then continuing my full walk is something I just don't do regularly. Here's my routine; while it is not absolutely proper, it works. I do an easy five-count stretch of three repetitions on each of the three primary muscle groups without a warm-up. It isn't as effective without the warm-up, but it helps some. I then take my exercise-walk and really get into the stretches after the walk, while my muscles are still warm. Getting the muscles stretched thoroughly at the end of your walk gives you the residual effect you want. If adequate time to stretch before and after walking is a problem, try to do one or the other—it is better than nothing.

Upper Body Stretches

Up until now, I have concentrated only on the muscles of the lower body. As you become an accomplished walker and start to pick up the pace, your upper body and arm swing will be increasingly important. You will need flexibility and looseness, particularly around the shoulder joints. This can be accomplished in the first 2 or 3 minutes of your walk.

As you begin your walk, loosen your arms and shoulders by swinging your arms across your body as if you were trying to wrap each one around your opposite side. Swing them with the right arm crossing over the left, then the left over the right. Swing them behind your back so that the fingers of the opposite hands touch. You will feel your back and shoulders loosen up after a few swings.

As you continue to walk, swing your arms around like windmills a few times, clockwise and counterclockwise. Nice, easy swings will loosen up the shoulder joints for a freer arm swing during your walk. Roll your head around clockwise and counterclockwise several times to loosen up your neck muscles. All of this can be done simultaneously with walking and warming up your leg muscles.

POSTURE, POSTURE, POSTURE

For exercise-walkers, proper posture is absolutely, positively, unequivocally, without a doubt the most critical, fundamental aspect of the walk. I can't say it with any more emphasis than that. Getting the body lined up properly before you take the first step and keeping it lined up through your entire walk will give you a more rewarding, less fatiguing workout. It will also help you improve your posture during your normal daily activities.

Why is correct posture so important? The American Physical Therapy Association has the best answer: "Good posture is important because it helps your body function at top speed. It promotes movement efficiency and endurance and contributes to an over-all feeling of well being." I can transfer all of this statement to walkers. I have observed that the slowest walkers (strollers) generally have the poorest posture, and the fastest walkers (race-walkers) have flawless posture.

Most strollers tend to walk with their heads tilted down, looking at the ground right in front of them. Their shoulders are slumped and their stomachs are sagging. Don't take my word for it; start your own observation of walkers' posture in relationship to their speed. You will find, as I did, that as the pace of the walk picks up, the requirement for good posture increases. Brisk walkers tend to have better posture than strollers. Aerobic walkers who are reaching for the 12-minute-mile pace just can't get there without good posture. Race-walkers, who require absolute "top speed" and "movement efficiency," walk with perfect posture. I have watched champion American race-walkers compete, and one thing they all have in common is perfect posture. They couldn't set records without it.

I realize that you are taking up exercise-walking not to set records but to improve your fitness and quality of life. According to the American Physical Therapy Association, "Good posture is also good prevention. . . . If you have poor posture, your bones are not properly aligned and your muscles, joints, and ligaments take more strain than nature intended. Faulty posture may cause you fatigue, muscular strain, and in later stages, pain."

One of the areas of discomfort when walking with bad posture is the lower back. Lower back pain rears its ugly head quickest for walkers with improper posture who are trying to increase their speed. When I had walkers in a clinic tell me that they get a pain in the lower back walking at a fast pace, I asked them to show me how they walk. Almost without exception they walked with the posture shown in Figure 5.8. Notice the vertical line of gravity and how the upper body is out in front of that line. The walker is increasing speed the wrong way: by literally falling forward. The walker releases good toning tension on the lower abdominal muscles and transfers it to the lower back muscles, where it shouldn't be. The back muscles have to work harder to hold the torso forward of the vertical line of gravity. Unnecessary fatigue ultimately becomes discomfort and pain in the lower back.

Let's get you properly lined up before you start your walking program. The alignment shown in Figure 5.9 is the one I used in my clinics, and it is recommended by the American Physical Therapy Association.

First, notice the vertical line of gravity. This imaginary line connects the ear, shoulder, hip, knee, and ankle. It also passes through the hypothetical center of mass (black square), which I added to the figure. In Figure 5.8 the head and entire upper body were tilted in front of the vertical line of gravity, causing the body to lurch forward by the pull of gravity instead of being powered forward by the big muscle groups in the legs.

Observe the spinal column in Figure 5.9. A properly aligned, healthy back has three natural curves: a slight forward curve in the neck (cervical curve), a slight backward curve in the upper back (thoracic curve), and a slight forward curve in the lower back (lumbar curve). The American Physical Therapy Associa-

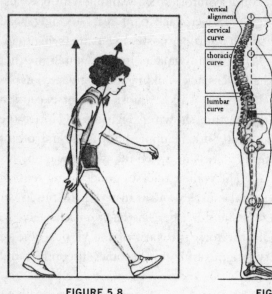

FIGURE 5.8

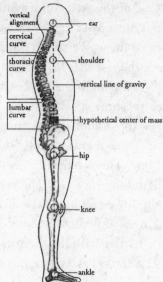

FIGURE 5.9

tion says, "Good posture actually means keeping these three curves in balanced alignment."

Putting the body in alignment is easy, but keeping it there is not, particularly if you aren't in shape or are considerably overweight. The muscles and joints are responsible for maintaining good posture. According to the American Physical Therapy Association, "Strong, flexible muscles are essential to good posture. Abdominal, hip, and leg muscles that are weak and inflexible cannot support your back's natural curves."

Your back's natural curves are balanced by your hip, knee, and ankle joints when you move about. Holding all of that in proper alignment while walking at a fast pace requires practice and perseverance, especially if you have had bad posture for

most of your life. I had a terrible time getting my posture together, and I confess that even today on a real fast walk I'll occasionally experience fatigue and discomfort in my lower back.
I check my posture, and sure enough, I am usually leaning forward a bit. It doesn't take much, and when I straighten up, the
discomfort goes away.

The way I used to teach posture was to start from the head
and go down, following the vertical line of gravity. Line yourself
up as in Figure 5.9, with a straight line through your ear, shoulder, hip, knee, and ankle. In the following illustrations you can
see how the imaginary vertical line of gravity relates to the front
and back view of someone with good posture. In the front view
(Figure 5.10A), the shoulders are of equal height, as are the hips
and knees. The head is held straight. The vertical line goes from
the point of the chin to the belly button and on down through the
center of the pelvis. In the view from the back (Figure 5.10B),
the spine and head are straight, not tilted or curved to the right
or left.

I have worked with enough people in walking clinics to
know that not everybody can have perfect posture, no matter
how hard they try. Some people have misalignments and variations in their musculoskeletal systems that do not result from
lack of effort on their part. Certainly some older people, especially women with osteoporosis, fall into that category.

Despite the changes that occur naturally with aging, good
posture can be maintained, and for many poor posture can be
improved. The American Physical Therapy Association advises:
"In individuals with severe postural problems, such as poor
alignments that have existed so long that structural changes
have occurred, the poor posture can be kept from getting
progressively worse." It recommends: "Everyone should con-

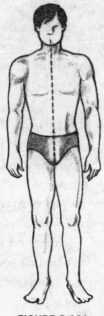 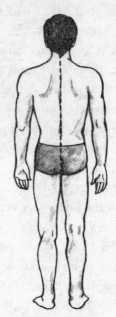

FIGURE 5.10A   **FIGURE 5.10B**

sciously work at achieving and maintaining good posture as they grow older." Baby boomers, listen up!

Now that you have seen what the elements of good posture are, here is a head-to-toe checklist:

- Head straight (not tilted to either side) with chin parallel to the ground
- Shoulders level and loose, in line with the ears and directly over the hips
- Chest held moderately elevated, with the upper back erect
- Hips level and directly under the shoulders
- Knees and ankles straight and in line with hips, shoulders, and ears

For those of you who have a posture problem, getting your head up and level and keeping it that way will be your biggest challenge. It was for me, and it was for most people in my clinics. Exercise-walkers tend to tilt their heads down and look almost straight down at the ground, as in Figure 5.11A.

The most common reason given for this position is, "I've got to see where I am going or I'll stumble." Sounds reasonable, but this really isn't the problem that everyone imagines. Take a look at runners; they are going much faster than walkers, yet you never see them with their heads down. Actually, it is difficult to run that way (try it). Runners' heads are up, and they are scanning the terrain ahead with their eyes. Walkers must learn to do the same.

You can see more than you think when you lower your eyes instead of your head. For instance, stand up now and put your head in the level position. Look across the room to the most distant point, as if you were scanning ahead of your walking path. Now scan with your eyes across the floor to see how close to your feet and line of travel you can see while keeping your chin parallel to the floor. Almost all people can see clearly to about 6 or 8 feet in front of them. That's really all the distance you need if you are constantly scanning ahead. Correct walking posture is shown in Figure 5.11B.

There is a fundamental reason to monitor your proper head position and to keep working on it until you can maintain it constantly. When the head tilts down, it tends to bring the shoulders with it, and then the back bends easily. The body tends to align itself from the top down. It is nearly impossible to have bad posture if your head is up and level. To prove this to yourself, stand up. With your head up and locked in the level position (ears in line with shoulders, chin parallel to the floor), see if you can slump your shoulders forward. As long as your head is

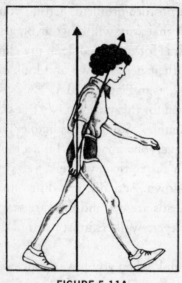

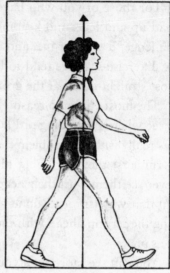

FIGURE 5.11A   **FIGURE 5.11B**

up and the cervical curve is locked, your shoulders and the rest of your body will stay in proper alignment. Good posture starts with the head.

THE STEP CYCLE AND ITS BIOMECHANICAL SUBTLETIES

Before we get into the stroll and its uses as a low-intensity exercise, a closer look at the walking gait will equip you to understand some of the less obvious biomechanical movements that occur on each step cycle. The more you understand your locomotion system and how it functions, the more you will appreciate what a complicated piece of biomechanical engineering you are. Everyone who owns a complex piece of high-tech equipment, or perhaps a well-engineered automobile, and who thoroughly understands and appreciates how it functions, will tend to use it and conscientiously maintain it. Perhaps when you know more about your body and its locomotion system, you will do likewise.

Over the years, I have looked for a well-researched book that examines the walking gait in minute detail. Dr. Lovejoy told me about such a book, appropriately entitled *Human Walking,* by Verne T. Inman, M.D., Ph.D.; Henry J. Ralston, Ph.D.; and Frank Todd. Dr. Inman was one of the pioneers in the use of electromyography (measuring the electric currents associated with muscular action) in the analysis of muscle function. The text of *Human Walking* is highly technical; it was written primarily for orthopedic doctors and other medical professionals. Nevertheless, I was able to mine a wealth of information out of it about the movements of our muscles and limbs during each step cycle: how our hips, shoulders, and legs rotate; how the foot and ankle move when we load our weight onto them; and what happens to all of these body parts when we introduce speed into our walking gait.

In the introduction Dr. Inman states, "The mastering of the erect bipedal type of locomotion is a relatively prolonged affair and appears to be a learned process, not the result of inborn reflexes." He compares a crawling infant with a quadruped as it uses one limb to advance and the other three as support. This tripod-type stability is lost when the infant tries to rise to a bipedal position and walk. Parents and grandparents marvel as the baby takes its first few unaided, faltering steps, and cringe with apprehension when it takes a few falls. As Dr. Inman points out, it is easy to observe that walking is a learning process for the baby. This does not seem to be true for the running gait, however. After slowly learning to walk, the young child quickly and instinctively learns how to run. We all have a survival instinct—fight or flight—and that is why I refer to running as our survival gait.

Because walking is a learned activity, it is not surprising that each of us has certain peculiarities in our walk. You can sometimes recognize a friend by his or her manner of walking, even from a great distance. The late John Wayne had a distinctive walk that was often imitated by impressionists. Dr. Inman observes: "Tall, slender people walk differently from short, stocky people and alter their manner of walking when wearing shoes with different heel heights." He also states, "A person walks differently when exhilarated than when mentally depressed," and concludes, "Any serious description of human walking should attempt an explanation of the dissimilarities as well as the similarities."

Upper body sway, for instance, varies with individuals. We all have this sway to some degree. It is caused by placing the lead foot wide from the track of the back foot at heel plant. As your weight is loaded onto that foot, you will list to that side. Babies learning to walk tentatively place their feet wide for stability and have a noticeable upper-body sway. We call them toddlers. If you are walking closely side by side with a friend and you are out of step, most likely your shoulders will bump because of upper body sway. Get in step and they won't bump, because you will both be swaying in the same direction at the same time. As you learn to increase your walking pace, you will find that excessive upper body sway is a hindrance.

According to Dr. Inman, the pelvis "becomes a suitable structure to separate the body into upper and lower parts which behave physically differently during walking." He points out that when walking at moderate speeds, "the pelvis lists, rotates, and undulates and the arms swing out of phase with the pelvis and legs." The upper and lower body rotate in different directions as our counterbalancing mechanism for stability. As Dr. Lovejoy pointed out, being upright and walking on two legs is biomechanically complex.

If you have ever walked behind someone in a pair of tight jeans, "pelvic rotation and undulation" probably became obvious. Dr. Inman observes that at a moderate pace your pelvis rotates approximately 4 degrees to either side of your vertical line of gravity. He adds, "As your speed increases, the pelvic rotation increases markedly." The pelvis does something else when you are walking: it lists downward on the side opposite the weight-bearing leg. The hardworking abductor muscles keep the body from tilting over when we became upright, but the body still has a list caused by the weight of the torso bearing down on the unsupported side. People who are extremely obese not only track wide for stability but also have considerable upper body sway and pelvic list as their locomotion system struggles to accommodate their excess weight.

Dr. Inman and his colleagues carefully researched the biomechanical subtleties of the human walking gait, which you will encounter as you learn about the various walking intensities. As Dr. Inman points out, "Every feature of walking changes when walking speed changes." Some of the movements of the limbs and muscles that function reasonably well at a slow pace take on different characteristics as the pace quickens. Being aware of this and understanding how to adjust for increased speed will help you become a smoother, better walker. Let's start slowly and work our way up:

STROLLING: LOW INTENSITY

You've stretched, you are standing erect with the proper posture, and you are ready to take the first step to start your lifetime exercise-walking program. I am purposely going to restate what I said in the previous chapter: in case you make mistakes when exercising, always err on the conservative side. Start slowly and avoid unnecessary discomfort; don't stress your cardiovascular system before it is ready.

If you start right, one of the many beauties of walking is that you can go from a sedentary, overweight lump all the way to a lean, mean race-walker (if that is your goal) without any soreness or injury. If you are in a totally unfit, sedentary condition, then you should definitely start at the strolling pace.

As stated in Chapter 4, the stroll is a low-intensity pace that ranges in speed from a 30-minute mile to an 18-minute mile. Within that range, you will automatically find a walking comfort zone. It will be determined by your age, state of unfitness, and how much excess weight you are carrying.

In the monthly walking clinics I conducted at the Cooper Wellness Program, I found that the older and heavier the walkers were, regardless of sex, the more slowly they had to start. For some a 30-minute mile was quite a challenge, and some couldn't go a mile at any pace. But that's okay. From that tortoise-like start, I have seen people combine desire with determination to achieve uncommon success. I enjoyed working with those slow starters because I remember when I was fat and sedentary. Don't be discouraged if you are in this condition. Desire, determination, and patience are far more important than speed at this stage.

Before you take your first step, let's establish what your

stride length should be. The definition of *stride* in the dictionary is "to walk with long steps." In common usage, however, when people say they were "striding along," they usually mean they were walking with some determination but with normal steps. Throughout the book, I also will use *stride* in this context.

The question of step or stride length came up in every one of my walking clinics, and there seemed to be differing opinions about it. The correct stride length for you is determined by the length of your legs, the length of your hamstrings, and the law of physics that governs a pendulum.

The femoral head of the upper leg is attached at the pelvis in a ball-and-socket arrangement. This is the pivotal point your leg swings from, and the length of your leg from there to the ground is the main determinant of your stride length. The leg swings back and forth like a pendulum—which it is. The law of physics that governs a pendulum says that long pendulums have longer arcs than short pendulums. It follows, then, that if you have long legs you will have a longer stride than someone with short legs. When dealing with the human body, however, there always seem to be exceptions, and there are a couple to this point. First, whatever degree of forward rotation you have in your pelvis will add to your stride length. For the stroll, brisk walk, or aerobic walk, let your pelvic rotation do what comes naturally. Do not try to exaggerate it. In Chapter 11 we will examine the effect of intentional forward pelvic flexion in race-walking.

Stride length can also be influenced by the hamstring muscles. They will keep your leg from swinging its normal arc if they are shorter than they should be. I can't say it often enough: muscles that aren't used lose their flexibility and functionality. This is especially true for people 50 and older. Because of short hamstrings, many older people walk with abnormally short strides;

some only shuffle. They can remedy this problem by regular stretching and regular walking.

There is an easy way for you to get an idea of what your stride length should be. Stand next to a wall or chair for balance, with all your weight on one leg. Tilt a bit toward your weight-bearing side so that your unweighted leg can clear the floor when it passes under your body. Hold your foot flat with your knee locked on the unweighted leg and let it swing freely in front of you, but don't force it forward. You will notice that your leg stops in front of you automatically and that it stops at about the same point every time. Now stop your leg at the exact end of its forward swing and slowly plant your heel on the ground as you push off with your other foot. If you don't have short ham-strings, this is your normal stride length. If you take a few steps of this length, they should feel comfortable and effortless.

To get a taste of what happens when you try to lengthen your stride beyond what it should be, repeat the foregoing pro-cedure, except force your leg beyond the point at which it auto-matically stops on the forward swing. Now slowly plant your heel and push off with your other foot. When the swing of your foot is forced beyond its normal arc, your center of mass will drop farther than it should because your foot is too far in front of you when it makes ground contact. This causes an exagger-ated, unrhythmic up-and-down action. Take a few steps like this and you can feel it. When exercise-walking, you are using your muscles and joints well within their normal range of mo-tion. Properly done, walking is a smooth, fluid, natural, rhyth-mic movement.

Before we leave the issue of stride length, let's put the big myth about tall people being able to walk faster than short peo-ple to rest once and for all. I wish I had a quarter for every time someone in my clinics has said to me, "Well, you can walk faster than I can because you're taller." If this were the case, Michael Jordan and Shaquille O'Neal could have been champion race-walkers as well as champion basketball players.

To resolve this old canard, we have to go back to physics class. The law governing pendulums says that long pendulums swing *slower* than short pendulums. It is true that someone 6 feet tall will have a longer stride length than someone 5 feet tall, but if both are of equal athletic ability, the 5-footer will be able to take more strides than the 6-footer. Walking speed is determined more by stride frequency than by stride length. Most of the world-champion men race-walkers are closer to 5 feet 9 inches than they are to 6 feet. Some of the champion women race-walkers are less than 5 feet tall but can walk faster than a 7-minute mile. I'll show you how to increase your stride frequency in the next chapter, but right now it's time to stroll.

Your Comfort Zone

The important thing for beginning exercise-walkers to remember is to let the walking gait find its own strolling comfort zone, which will vary with the individual. Some people starting from sedentary can tolerate more exercise sooner than others. This can be a problem for husbands and wives, friends, or neighbors who want to start a walking program together. If both are sedentary but one is just a little overweight and the other is extremely overweight, the lighter walker may be comfortable at a 20-minute-mile pace while the heavier walker struggles to keep up. The danger in this situation is that the overweight walker may be putting too much stress on his or her cardiovascular system. It is also counterproductive for the faster walker to reduce the intensity of his or her walk for a slower walker.

By definition, strolling is a low-intensity physical exercise.

Even so, I have worked with many people who felt as if they were climbing Pike's Peak as they struggled through their first mile in 25 or 30 minutes. If you are at this level, just hang in there and keep plugging away, because I have also had the pleasure of seeing those people cruising along at a brisk 15-minute-mile pace a few months later. Find your own comfort zone and stay with it until you improve your level of fitness. Above all, don't try to keep up with a faster walker until you are physically ready. The stroll is the entry-level walk for people with great variations of unfitness.

Strolling Objectives

Your two primary objectives with the strolling pace are, in order of importance, to achieve your goal for frequency and to achieve your goal for duration in terms of either minutes or miles. Intensity of exercise is not a consideration with the stroll, even though a walker who is struggling along at a 30-minute mile may think the 20-minute stroll is light-years away. I can assure this walker that he or she will see the day when the 20-minute mile not only isn't a challenge but may actually be boring, as our strollers in the walking study found. If this occurs, all you have to do is pick up the pace a bit. Happily, at that point your body will be ready for the increased physical challenge.

Work on your frequency and duration together—but slowly. If five days a week is your goal—and it's a good one—try to get in a little walk each day. It is better to go often for short walks than infrequently for long ones. Frequency adds to your discipline, and the sooner you make time every day for your walk, the sooner you will be on your way to an increased quality of life.

I vividly remember trying to make this point about walking every day in a walking clinic by comparing it to the need to brush our teeth every day. I feel so strongly about the merits of exercise-walking and the physical evils of being sedentary that in my lectures I sometimes paced back and forth and became almost evangelistic. On this particular day, I stopped, planted my feet, gave the class a hellfire-and-brimstone look, and with a demanding voice asked, "Would any of you even *think* of going a day without brushing your teeth?" An old guy off to my left got up, pulled out his uppers and lowers, and with a gummy smile waved them at me and the class. I went to my knees laughing, and a middle-aged woman next to him laughed so hard, she lost control of her bladder. Believe me, I'll never forget that clinic.

The stroll is the perfect pace to help you reach your duration goal. Three miles a day, which was recommended by the President's Council on Physical Fitness, is the goal I think is the most sustainable and effective over the long term. Covering this distance at a stroll, particularly a slow stroll, takes considerable time. But in the early stages of your walking program, you must allow for it so that you don't overload your physiological system. Once you can do 3 miles at a comfortable strolling pace, you'll be ready to work on intensity.

In addition to reaching your frequency and duration goals with the stroll, you should use this pace to establish firmly the proper walking posture. Most slow walkers tend to amble along in a slouched posture. Once your fitness improves and your initial slow pace is no longer a physical challenge, you will naturally want to increase your speed—and you should. The faster you walk, however, the more important correct posture becomes. The stroll is the ideal pace to put good walking habits in place.

I find that the tendency to tilt the head downward and slump the shoulders is the most difficult bad posture habit to break. Until you get your proper walking posture firmly in place, say to yourself, "Hips forward, shoulders back, chin up . . . hips forward, shoulders back, chin up . . . hips forward, shoulders back, chin up." Repeat that in cadence with your steps. As you walk faster, speed it up and repeat it over and over like a mantra. You will probably find that correcting a downward tilted head is your biggest posture problem. Work on it. If I can do it, *anyone* can do it.

One final thing: don't walk with your hands in your pockets. Let them hang loose at your sides and swing back and forth freely in a relaxed manner. You don't have to swing them vigorously when strolling; that comes later. The arms counterbalance your leg and pelvic movements, however, and add to the rhythm of your walk. The stroll is the most accommodating pace to practice your posture, technique, and rhythm. When you've got all of that together and have hit your goals for frequency and duration, you are ready to move up to the brisk pace.

SIX

Brisk Walking and Aerobic Walking

BRISK WALKING

The brisk walk—18- to 14-minute miles—is the pace that most long-term exercise-walkers use. It delivers enough cardiovascular improvement and caloric expenditure for the time spent to be the best all-around exercise. On a risk-reward basis for all people who do not have a physical impairment in their walking gait, it can't be beat.

Dr. Kenneth Cooper believes that the importance of consistency in exercise is far greater than intensity. The preoccupation with intensity of exercise since fitness awareness began about thirty years ago has turned many people off. As I mentioned earlier, high-impact aerobics is a dead issue, and the jogging craze has leveled off. Dr. Cooper, one of the earliest proponents of jogging and running, now firmly says, "Walk more, run less."

Intensity is still a major factor, however, in any exercise or training program. But we now know that the intensity of exercise an individual needs for a meaningful contribution to his or her cardiovascular fitness, health, and quality of life is much less than an athlete needs when training for a specific sport. The brisk pace fulfills this intensity need beautifully.

The brisk pace is rated as a moderate-intensity exercise, and because of this it has great sustainability for people of all ages—even some in their eighties. Equally important, it delivers an adequate amount of *perceived exertion* for most people. By that I mean that brisk walkers feel physically and mentally challenged enough that they do not become bored. Each walk is a rewarding experience for mind and body. If you recall in Chapter 4, Dr. Duncan had to put down a minor revolt with some of our 20-minute-mile strollers in the walking study because their walks became monotonous. They were no longer physically and mentally challenged by the strolling pace. Conversely, we didn't have any complaints from the 15-minute-mile brisk walkers.

Arm Swing

To move up to the brisk pace, an exercise-walker must become aware of the importance of the role that the arm swing plays in accelerating the walking gait. It is easy to walk at the strolling pace with one's arms totally inactive; however, you should not walk with them in your pockets. Walking with your hands in your pockets limits your ability to increase your pace.

Just like the legs, the arms are compound pendulums, and

their pivotal points are the shoulders. The arms as pendulums also have a natural arc to their swing, depending on their length from the shoulder joint to the hand. Knowing how to implement a coordinated arm swing with an increased leg swing becomes important from this point on—especially if you want to move beyond the brisk walking pace.

To check your arm swing, stand up and assume the correct posture, with your feet directly under your hips. With your shoulders relaxed and your arms hanging loosely at your sides, notice that they don't hang straight; there is a slight bend at the elbow. Swing your arms back and forth, alternating the right and left arms as if you were walking, but keep them rigid at the elbow so there is no forearm flop. Hold the arm rigid from your shoulder to your hand as if it were one long bone. Get a full, vigorous swing, but don't try to force either arm beyond the point that feels natural, especially on the front swing.

If you swing your arms for a few seconds, you will develop a rhythm and a distance of travel on the front and back swing that feels as if each arm is in a groove. You will see that your arm on the front swing stops at about the same point every time. The same is true on the back swing. Your arm pendulum has found its arc of travel, based on the length of the arm, and to some extent the looseness and flexibility of your shoulder joint and arm muscle attachments.

When you stop your arm at the end of its arc on the front swing, notice that it has come slightly *across* your body. It should not, however, come across your vertical line of gravity (the hypothetical line from your chin down through your navel and the center of your pelvis). If it does, you will be getting too much sideways motion, which distorts the arm swing's counterbalancing role relative to the legs.

I have observed some people who swing their arms straight

out, parallel to their leg swing. This has an artificial, military look to it. Such an arm swing may work for the stroll and brisk paces, but, as you will find out later in this chapter, it will definitely limit your ability to accelerate beyond the brisk pace, if that is your goal. Try to find that groove where your arm comes slightly across your body but not across your vertical line of gravity.

You probably have not paid much attention to the biomechanics of your walking gait up until now—at least most people haven't. Whether you have noticed it or not, your arms alternate with your legs on each step when you walk fast. For example, as your right leg swings forward, your left arm swings forward and vice versa. How much the arm swing actually contributes to forward propulsion will be discussed in detail later in the chapter. For now, I will let you find out for yourself that a good, vigorous arm swing helps you move along smartly.

On your next walk, pick a point about 40 yards away, put your hands in your pockets (preferably pants pockets, as opposed to jacket pockets), and see how fast you can comfortably and rhythmically walk the distance. Then take your hands out of your pockets and, with your arms swinging fully extended and vigorously as you have just practiced, see how fast you can walk back. There will be a significant difference in the rhythm of your walk and your ability to walk faster with seemingly less effort. From now on your arm swing becomes an important ally to your leg swing as you attempt to increase the pace of your walk.

We have established what your natural stride length and your natural arm swing should be. As a brisk walker, you now put them together, and the faster you make your arms and legs swing, the faster you go. Your increased pace should be smooth, rhythmic, and comfortable. Don't force a fast pace by losing your erect posture or by excessive arm swing that isn't in sync with your leg swing. The minute you start to feel awkward, slow down, relax a bit, and smooth out your walk, then gradually pick up the pace again.

Straight-Leg Swing

A nice, rhythmic walking style with a low center of gravity and proper posture is the technique you want for the brisk pace. When your swing leg comes forward, it should be fully extended and straight at the knee as the heel is placed on the ground. When your back foot pushes off and forces your body forward over that leg, keep it straight as it passes under you and becomes the trailing leg. The proper technique is shown in Figure 6.1.

In Figure 6.1A, the walker is in the double-stance phase, that brief moment when the front heel has made contact with the ground and the back toe has not yet left the ground. Notice that the lead leg is completely straight at the knee. Notice also that it is still straight at the knee as it passes under the body in Figure 6.1B.

Some people tend to walk with high bent-knee action on their lead leg. This causes them to land on the sole of their foot and to bob up and down. If they try to walk fast in this manner, they do more bobbing than going forward. If their knee is bent when it passes under them, they have that old Groucho Marx look, as if they were doing a fast creep.

Chances are your leg is fairly straight at heel plant and as it passes under your body. Some people, however, as they start to walk faster, tend to pick up speed by bending the knees. This happens most often as walkers try to move up to the aerobic pace. If you see people walking fast—or attempting to—with

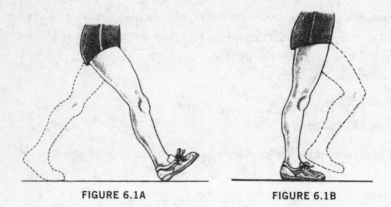

FIGURE 6.1A   **FIGURE 6.1B**

their knees bent, they are probably doing a light flat-footed jog instead of a fast walk. Their locomotion system is using more elastic energy from their muscles instead of the lifting and falling mechanical energy of their leg pendulums. They are using a sort of hybrid gait that denies them the best benefits of either a good run or a fast walk. Check your leg swing and work on keeping your leg straight through the entire step cycle, from heel plant to weight bearing to toe-off.

Heel Plant to Toe-Off

As the heel makes contact with the ground, the forefoot and toes should be up at a comfortable angle (see Figure 6.2). Bringing the toes up at heel plant eliminates landing on the sole of the foot and clumping along in an awkward manner. In addition to stride length and the straight-leg swing, the way you load your body weight onto your foot after heel plant will determine how smooth and rhythmic your walk will be. As the foot is lowered after heel plant, it should not slap down flat from heel to toe but

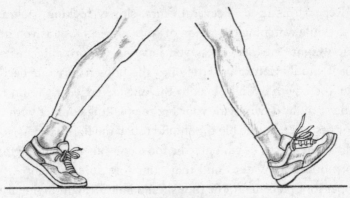

FIGURE 6.2

should settle in smoothly with a slight emphasis on the outside (lateral) edge.

Here is an experiment that will clearly show you how your foot functions as you put your weight on it in a walking step. If you aren't at home as you are reading this, you may have to wait until you get there to try this experiment.

Take off your shoe and sock on one foot. For balance, it might be best to stand next to a chair. Put your sockless foot out in front of you with your heel on the floor and your toes up as if you had just taken a step and made floor contact at heel plant. Have your other foot slightly behind you, flat on the floor and bearing weight. Now slowly elevate the heel of your back foot, as if you are starting to toe off. Let your front foot settle onto the floor gently and naturally until it is flat and you have transferred all of your weight on it. Keep the toes of your back foot in contact with the floor. Reverse and transfer your weight onto your back foot again by letting the heel settle back down onto the floor as your front toes rise to their original position.

Repeat this process several times, slowly rocking back and forth while watching the action of your sockless foot as you load your weight onto it. Unless you have an abnormality in your foot it should naturally settle onto the floor from your heel to your toes, with a slight bias to the outside edge. It should not come straight down, with your big toe making contact with the floor first. In fact, the big toe should touch the floor last. As your full weight comes down onto the foot, you can see that the fore-foot noticeably widens and that your toes spread slightly. For proper foot placement, the foot should land straight in line from heel plant to toe-off. Some people have their toes pointed in at toe-off—a condition commonly referred to as being "pigeon-toed." Others walk with one or both feet splaying out from their line of travel.

By the time people reach adulthood, they will probably walk the rest of their lives the way that their feet are presently tracking. Most have adapted to it and do quite well. In my clinics I didn't try to change the way they plant their feet because, as Dr. Inman points out, "There are great dissimilarities in the walking gait." You should know, however, that foot placement that deviates from proper alignment (whether the toes point in or out) will affect your ability to increase your pace. Someone who toes in or splays out noticeably may find it difficult to walk at a brisk pace.

By now you are probably wondering how you are going to remember all the nuances involved with something supposedly as simple as walking. It will be easier than you think. I suspect you are probably not very far off on many of them. In my clinics I found that most people had pretty good technique and only needed to brush up on a point or two.

When something you are doing almost unconsciously is broken down biomechanically, it sometimes seems to become mentally and physically complicated. A few people put too much thought into it and try to micromanage their walking gait. That usually leads to a stiff, unrelaxed walker. Get out, start walking, and check yourself out; you may be a natural, and if so, all you have to do is keep going.

In order of importance, you should concentrate on (1) posture, (2) technique (leg stride and foot action), and (3) rhythm. Try to develop a fluid, smooth gait. Observe other walkers. You will see great variations of the walking gait—some people with heads bobbing up and down, others seeming to lurch from side to side. Then you will see a walker who moves with it all together in one coordinated, flowing stride.

Starting with the stroll and working up to the fast end of the brisk pace, a sedentary person can develop a good, moderate level of fitness—and this is all many people need or want. Others, however, want the benefits of an aerobic workout, and they are willing to put the necessary intensity into their exercise to achieve the higher aerobic fitness level.

The top end of the brisk pace is subaerobic for a fit individual. Consequently, most people are told to switch to another form of exercise, such as running, to get the intensity necessary to attain aerobic fitness or to accelerate caloric expenditure. As you learned in Chapter 4, this is no longer necessary. Aerobic walking can take you as far up the fitness ladder as you want to go.

AEROBIC WALKING

Aerobic walking involves making one simple change in your arm swing that enables you to accelerate your walk from the brisk 15-minute-mile pace to a 12-minute mile or faster. The results are spectacular for weight loss, cardiovascular fitness, stress relief, and increased energy. By walking aerobically, you'll burn as many calories as a jogger and get a complete head-to-toe workout. Aerobic walking uses all the major muscle groups in the upper and lower body in a low-impact, dynamic, rhythmic action, which is exactly what an ideal exercise should do.

Aerobic walking is a high-intensity exercise, but one you can engage in without the concern for injury that goes with many other high-intensity exercises, such as running. When my first walking book was completed, I had an obvious choice for a title. Since it focused on walking at a pace that would put your heart into the recognized aerobic-training range, and since aerobic exercise is so widely recommended, it seemed to make sense to call it *Aerobic Walking*. This designation also helps to simplify identifying the other walking intensity levels.

High-intensity aerobic walking is easily distinguished from the moderate and low intensities of brisk walking and strolling. Aerobic walking's pace is equal to slow jogging, and an altered arm swing is required to walk this fast. Confusion seems to arise when one deviates from what is perceived as normal walking, and too many in the fitness field are apt to call any such change "race-walking." Since race-walking is not well understood or widely viewed as a major track-and-field event in this country, some people shy away from altering their walking form. In Chapter 11 I will cover all the adjustments to the walking gait required for one to become a competitive race-walker.

I learned the race-walking technique when I was researching my first book and assumed it was required to achieve a walking pace fast enough to get an aerobic workout. That is not the case. The experience of working with thousands of people in walking clinics over many years has proven to me that one simple change of the arm swing is all that is necessary to accelerate your walking speed from a brisk pace to an aerobic 12-minute mile or faster. This is what I taught the women aerobic walkers in the walking study in Chapter 4. They walked magnificently, and many hit the upper end (86 percent) of their aerobic training range consistently.

The Bent-Arm-Swing Technique

Perhaps the most difficult message to get across in a walking clinic is the relative importance of a vigorous bent-arm swing to increase walking speed. It raises this question: if the walking-propulsion muscles are in the legs, then how do the arms make you go faster? When stride frequency is increased, the arm swing (in its counterbalancing role) must increase also. If the arms do not keep up with the legs, the entire walking gait becomes out of sync and labored; speed is then difficult, if not impossible, to achieve and maintain.

Dr. Inman states: "Walking is a complex integrated activity with multiple factors interacting simultaneously." This truism takes on new meaning as you try to increase your walking speed. The interaction of the arms and legs becomes more apparent. The biomechanical role the arms play in walking at a stroll is minimal. At that pace, you can even walk comfortably with your hands in your pockets. If you took the 40-yard walking test earlier in this chapter and tried to walk fast that way, you found that doing so not only was uncomfortable but actually restricted your ability to stride out at a faster pace.

Walking at the brisk pace with the arms fully extended and swinging freely at your sides, it is easy to get a smooth, comfortable leg swing and to maintain your speed. The brisk pace tops out at about a 14-minute mile, however, or at least becomes so labored that it is uncomfortable to maintain because your fully extended arms cannot swing fast enough to serve as counterbalancers.

When you are walking at a pace that is equivalent to a slow jog, your arms must be able to swing fast enough to complement and counterbalance the increased leg swing. The long, extended-arm pendulum must be shortened so that you can swing it faster. The compound feature of your arm pendulum permits you to bend it at the elbow and bring the forearm up so that it forms a 90-degree angle with your upper arm. In effect, you have shortened your arm so that you can swing it faster. By locking the angle at the elbow so that your forearm does not flop up and down, you allow it to swing in a natural arc. Discounting the slight effect of the weight of the forearm, your arms are essentially swinging pendulums as long as the distance from the bottom of your elbow to your shoulder joint. The shortened arm pendulums will now swing as fast as you can make your legs go.

A way to feel the difference in swing frequency is to stand with one arm fully extended and locked rigid at the elbow. Swing your long-arm pendulum back and forth as fast as you can within its normal swing range. Don't swing it on the forward swing any farther than you would when walking briskly.

Now bring your forearm up to a 90-degree angle at the elbow and pump your upper arm back and forth as fast as you can. Notice how much faster it swings. A metronome, used by musicians to maintain a beat, works the same way. With the weight farthest from the point of swing it goes slowest, but as the weight is moved closer to the point of swing, the beat goes faster.

Your forearm, wrist, and hand hanging down fully extended

put most of the weight of your arm *below* the elbow. This makes your arm act like the slow metronome. The simple act of elevating this weight, even with the elbow, permits your arms to swing faster.

If you have progressed through the frequency, duration, and intensity sectors of your walking program and can walk 3 miles in 45 minutes without undue physical stress, you are a prime candidate for aerobic walking. You have achieved a moderate level of fitness and are already contributing to your health, to your quality of life, and possibly to your longevity.

Walking faster will increase your cardiovascular fitness, which will give you a decrease in resting heart rate, an increase in maximal oxygen consumption (VO_2 max), and the ability to accomplish a given task at a lower percentage of VO_2 max. Simply stated, aerobic walking will make your heart more fit to function at a high level and enable you to engage in more physical activities with less fatigue.

I walk aerobically every day even at my advanced age, as does my 67-year-old wife, and we find it the perfect aerobic exercise. It is a quick way to burn extra calories, and the increased cardiovascular fitness from it gives us a higher energy level. The intensity component of exercise-walking, however, should be added only if you can consistently maintain frequency and duration. *If you are under a doctor's care, it is important that he or she concurs.* If you are game and have tagged all of those bases, then let's give it a whirl.

Some interesting things happen to some people when they start to walk fast with their arms bent at the elbow. Everyone has heard the old saw about people who are "so uncoordinated they can't walk and chew gum at the same time." Don't laugh; you might feel like this yourself for a bit. You have walked your whole life, your arms flopping along at your sides, without thinking about them. Now, with them bent, some people start to think about their arms—and sometimes strange things happen.

When the mind begins to manage the arms, which it has paid no attention to up until now, there is a tendency to swing an arm forward on the same side as the leg that is swinging forward. This creates a stilted, uncoordinated look. The walker immediately senses something is wrong but can't quite figure out what.

Men are probably tired of hearing me rave about women's walking competence, but, in most of the classes I have taught, more men than women have trouble with the bent-arm swing. At the Cooper Wellness Program, where the average age of the participants was 48, I found that a number of middle-aged men tended to walk like the Energizer bunny, while their wives were cruising around the track like sports cars.

Generally, the bent-arm swing is only a temporary problem, but with humans there always seems to be exceptions. In 1989, I had a 42-year-old investment banker from Illinois named Larry in a walking clinic. When he used the bent-arm swing and walked, his knees came up as if he were a drum major marching. When I had him drop his forearms to their natural position, his knees went down to their natural position. Larry walked as if he had strings connecting his wrists to his knee caps. When a wrist went up, so did the knee. He was still fighting his problem when we parted later that day. Larry is the only person I know who couldn't master the bent-arm swing in a short time.

Before you attempt to change to the bent-arm swing on your daily walk, try a little coordinating experiment at home. Stand with your head up, chin parallel to the floor, and posture erect as if you were walking, except keep your feet stationary directly under your pelvis. Let your shoulders relax and let your arms swing fully extended and vigorously, as if you were on a brisk walk. Swing them through their full normal range from front to back.

On the front swing you will notice that just as the upper arm stops its motion the forearm will continue upward and slightly across your body by bending at the elbow from the momentum of the swing. Swing the arms several times so that you are relaxed at the shoulders.

Now, while swinging the arms, slowly raise the forearms until they are at right angles to your upper arms. Keep the shoulders relaxed; some people tend to elevate their shoulders when they elevate their forearms. Keep swinging the arms, then lower them to the extended position again. Repeat this cycle several times to see if you are equally relaxed at the shoulders whether your forearms are up or down. Sometimes, as the swing frequency is increased, coordination suffers and tightness in the shoulders develops. When you feel as relaxed and coordinated with the forearms up as down, increase the frequency of their swing to see how fast you can move them back and forth.

I find it is easier for most people to get the hang of the bent-arm swing by swinging their arms while standing—preferably in front of a mirror—than when out walking. If you swing them properly, the upper arms will not travel any farther than they did when the arms were fully extended. However, because the forearm now projects in front of you, it seems as if the upper arm does go farther.

To prove that the upper arm travels the same distance, in my clinics I used to put a Day-Glo orange armband around my elbow to focus attention on the length of the arc it travels while the arm is swinging fully extended. As I raise my forearm to the 90-degree angle, the arc of the swing remains exactly the same.

If the forearm is not brought all the way up to a 90-degree angle, you are swinging a partially shortened pendulum that will put some drag on your ability to achieve the maximum frequency of your arm swing. Many people tend to let their forearms hang below their elbows. It is always better to bend the forearm a little bit above the elbow than to let it hang below.

With the forearm in its new position, a couple of tendencies occur in most people's arm swings. One is to swing the arms too high on the front swing and not far enough on the back swing. Figure 6.3 shows the arm in its proper position at the end of the front swing.

Let your hand form a loose fist with your thumb resting on the first joint of your forefinger. If you clench your fist, you will tighten the muscles in the arm and become tense. The arms should hang loosely from the shoulders so that the forearms and elbows pass close to your body. If you are wearing a sweatshirt or jacket, it is okay for the sleeve to brush your body lightly. At the end of the front swing, your hand should be slightly across the front of your body, but not across the center line of gravity as shown in Figure 6.3, and the hand should never go higher than the line across the top of your breast.

On the back swing, your loose fist should come to about the middle of your buttocks, as in Figure 6.4. Most people tend to stop short on the back swing. Try bringing your loose fist back to just behind the seam of your pants and you will probably feel a slight pull at your shoulder. Hold your loose fist still at your hip at the end of its back-swing arc for a couple of seconds, then quickly relax the shoulder muscles. The shortened arm pendulum will naturally drop forward, and it only takes a little muscle power to increase the speed of its forward swing. Concentrate on putting muscle power into your back swing. If your arm pen-

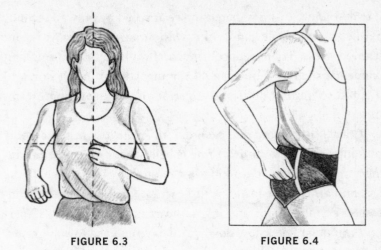

FIGURE 6.3   FIGURE 6.4

dulum gets a full, vigorous back swing, the front swing will almost take care of itself.

I promise you that if you couple correct posture with your normal stride length and the bent-arm-swing technique, you can rise to the top end of your aerobic training range. You do not have to change the normal way your legs and hips move. This is not race-walking; it is aerobic walking. Coordinate your faster bent-arm swing with your faster leg swing and take off.

MOVE FROM BRISK TO AEROBIC WALKING—SLOWLY

I don't want to leave you with the impression that if you simply bend your arms and swing them a little faster you will automatically go from a brisk 15-minute mile to an aerobic 12-minute mile. More important, you should not even try to do so. Pick up the pace a little at a time. If you are now walking 3 miles in 45 minutes, see if the new arm-swing technique will help you to do it in 44 minutes. That's increasing your speed by only 20 seconds a mile. Most people can do this without any discomfort or unwanted stress. Try to reduce your total walking time in small increments, such as 3 miles in 44 minutes, down to 43, down to 42, and so on, but do it over a period of weeks or months, not days.

Check your heart rate each day to see if it is in the aerobic training range. If your heart rate is below your 65 percent training range, you aren't walking fast enough to be aerobic. If the legs and arms move faster, your heart rate will automatically increase. Equally important: if your heart rate is over your 85 percent training range, slow down. You have no need to walk faster. Your heart rate is telling you that your fitness level isn't as good as you think it is. For instance, if walking a 14-minute mile puts your heart rate over 85 percent, then increasing your speed would be a mistake. You should actually slow down a little. As your fitness level rises, your heart rate will decline; *then* you can pick up the pace of your walk. Remember: *heart rate is always more important than minutes per mile as a gauge of your fitness level*. This is why I suggest that you invest in a heart rate monitor.

DOMINANT- AND SUBDOMINANT-ARM SWING

The bent-arm swing's contribution to an exercise-walker's ability to increase walking speed to a 12-, 11-, or even 10-minute mile cannot be overstated. Without it, your pace will plateau. To get the maximum benefit, the arms must swing in the groove shown in Figures 6.3 and 6.4. For the arms to be fully effective as counterbalances for the legs, they should also swing *evenly*.

It is an unusual person who can move to the bent-arm swing

with the swing in both the right and left arms evenly matched. By this I mean that a person who is right-handed will have a more coordinated, vigorous swing with his or her right arm (the dominant arm) than with the left (the subdominant). Of course, the reverse is also true. I am a lefty, so my right arm is the one that requires my concentration. I used to have fun in my clinics telling participants whether they are right- or left-handed simply by watching their bent-arm swing. The dominant and subdominant difference is more difficult to call when the arm is fully extended. I asked people to bend their arms and pump them back and forth as if they were walking. The most obvious tip-off to the subdominant arm is that the person does not take it as far back on the back swing as the dominant arm or as far forward on the front swing. It swings midrange in a namby-pamby manner and the elbow is usually away from the rib cage. People are often amazed at the difference between their arm swings.

You can check the difference on yourself. Place your subdominant hand firmly on the point of your dominant shoulder just above where the upper arm joins the shoulder. For example, right-handers would place their left hand on their right shoulder, and southpaws would do the opposite. Now pump the dominant arm vigorously back and forth as if you were doing the bent-arm swing. Take it clear back to the middle of the buttocks and as far forward as shown in Figure 6.3. After pumping it a few times to feel the coordinated vigor of the swing, reverse the procedure. With your dominant hand on your subdominant shoulder, pump this arm the same way. I have had people laugh out loud when their subdominant arm swung out where they didn't want it to go. They couldn't believe that there could be so much variance in the coordination of their arms. You may not have a lot of variance, but I suspect there will be enough to notice some difference in vigor and coordination between your arms.

This dominant-subdominant difference in arm swing is a subtlety you should be aware of so that you can continually monitor your subdominant arm to make sure you are getting a balanced arm swing. As you pick up your walking speed, it becomes more critical that each part of your musculoskeletal system be coordinated and balanced in every phase of each step cycle. If you decide to progress to race-walking, a balanced arm swing is a must. It takes awhile to get consistent balance in the arm swing, and even then there will be lapses.

Those of you with video cameras, have someone tape your various walking intensities. This is an excellent way to check the progress of your walking form for posture, arm swing, foot placement, and leg action.

THE ARM-SWING DRILL

To establish the importance of the relationship of arm swing and leg speed, I used to run a little drill in my clinics that required the participants to set the pace of their walk with their *arms* instead of their legs. As participants went a distance no longer than a basketball court, I would get next to the walkers and keep repeating, "Pump your arms, pump your arms," to get them to move their arms as fast as they could while trying to keep their legs moving in sync.

When a walker gets his arms and legs moving in synchrony and sets the cadence of the walk by pumping the arms fast, the legs want to follow. In fact, the arms can pump so fast that the legs will want to break into a jog. There seems to be a neuro-motor connection between your arms and legs that makes them want to work in unison at high speed.

As part of the arm-swing drill, I also had people walk as fast as they could for about half the distance of a basketball court using the bent-arm swing. When they were in full stride and halfway across, I would shout, "Drop them," and have them drop their forearms quickly to the fully extended position and swing them as fast as they could while continuing to walk quickly. I generally heard a few loud groans and saw a few smiles as the walkers felt the drag of the fully extended arm pendulum. As one woman said, "My God, it's like dropping an anchor!" Try it yourself; you'll feel it too.

In addition to helping you walk faster, the bent-arm swing has another little plus. Many who walk several miles at a brisk pace with their arms fully extended and swinging vigorously complain of fingers swelling—sometimes so much so that the area around a ring can become painful. This pooling of blood and fluids in the fingers and hands caused by the centrifugal force of the extended arm does not occur with the bent-arm swing.

Once the forearm is brought up into the 90-degree position, it is important to keep the wrist and hand in line with the arm. Some people—women more than men—tend to let their hands flop up and down, as in Figure 6.5A. The correct position is shown in Figure 6.5B. A flopping movement at the end of the forearm transfers up the arm and affects the arm swing.

When you master the bent-arm swing and get your dominant and subdominant arms swinging with equal vigor, the only limits on how fast you can walk will be determined by your ability to maintain concentration. As your walking speed progresses beyond the 14-minute mile, you will find that if your mind wanders, your speed will drop. This is a common experience as people increase their walking speed into the range of a slow jog. Over time, the amount of concentration needed diminishes, but it still remains more than is required for jogging.

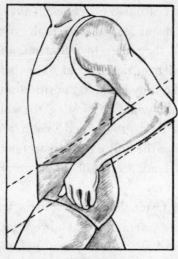

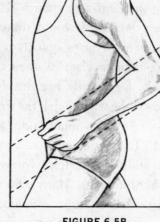

FIGURE 6.5A   FIGURE 6.5B

Walking at the aerobic pace becomes a physical *and* mental exercise because it requires a rhythmic coordination of your upper and lower body, plus the mental concentration to force your pace beyond a normal brisk walk. Jogging is a no-brainer exercise, but I don't mean that in a derogatory way. Find out for yourself. Walk as fast as you can for about 40 yards, then kick into a jog at the same pace and see how it requires less concentration and physical effort. Now drop back to a walk at the same pace as the jog. You will immediately recognize that an aerobic walk is far more challenging, both physically and mentally, than jogging at the same pace. Running is our survival gait, so it makes sense that you shouldn't have to think about it. After all, if you are running for your life, you already have enough on your mind.

As testimony to the perceived difference in exertion between aerobic walking and jogging, I had to smile when I received a letter from Dr. Kenneth Cooper on a matter not related to walking. In a postscript he wrote, "I have been experimenting with race-walking [he really meant aerobic walking] myself! I am now able to walk 5 kilometers [3.1 miles] averaging faster than 12 minutes per mile. For a 'confirmed runner' that is a fast walk!" You bet it is, and all runners, "confirmed" or otherwise, struggle when they try to walk fast. Dr. Cooper was referring to aerobic walking as race-walking, but this is a common mistake, and I will clear up the confusion between the two in Chapter 11.

Some walkers—women more than men—find that their upper arms tire when they convert to the bent-arm swing. The combination of swinging the arms faster and holding the forearms up temporarily causes biceps fatigue. If this occurs, just lower your forearms enough to relieve the fatigue. After you have rested them awhile, pull them up to the 90-degree angle again until they tire. Keep repeating this fatigue-and-rest cycle during your walk, and in a few days the fatigue will be gone.

One final comment about bent arms. The first thing runners do is pull their arms up to a 90-degree angle. Do you ever see distance runners or exercise joggers with their arms hanging at their sides fully or even partially extended? Because runners are bouncing along with the elastic energy from their leg muscles, their arms have no role in their propulsion. Even so, runners couldn't run very fast if their arms were hanging down at their sides. Try it sometime. Walkers can't walk very fast either with their arms fully extended at their sides. Aerobic walkers (and race-walkers) must use their arms in a stride-for-stride vigorous pumping action, much the way sprinters do.

THE 13-MINUTE-MILE WALL

Since my book *Aerobic Walking* was published, I have gotten a good number of letters and phone calls from people who say they are using the bent-arm-swing technique but they just can't get beyond a 13-minute mile. In walking clinics that I have conducted from Boston to San Diego, the 13-minute-mile wall seems to stop a lot of aerobic walkers temporarily. To get through it becomes a matter of mind over muscle.

Once you get your arms and legs working in synchrony, the next challenge is to get your brain to signal your leg muscles to move as fast as you want them to. In the normal range of walking that is not a problem, but walking faster than a 13-minute mile is well beyond the normal range. The walking muscles must be programmed to fire at that intensity. The brain sends a signal out to the muscles, which are to perform a certain function, and electrical impulses within the muscles fire. The muscles then perform their specific function. For instance, make a fist and then open and close your fist as fast as you can, a few times. That happened because your brain was sending a signal out to fire the muscles in your hand to make them contract and relax as you wanted.

I find the many similarities between our biomechanical locomotion system and the automobile fascinating. I told you about the similarities of gaits to gears in Chapter 2. There is also a similarity between the muscles firing by electrical impulse to move the body about and the spark plugs in a car's motor firing an electrical spark to make the fuel explode and power the pistons, which make the driveshaft and ultimately the car move.

The brain signals the muscles to get them to move by way of motor neurons. (The dictionary defines *motor neuron* as "a nerve cell that conducts impulses to a muscle.") In their book on human walking, Dr. Inman and associates state, "The response of muscles in the body depends on several factors: (1) The number of motor neurons activating the muscle at any given moment, and (2) The rates at which the various motor neurons are firing." If you want to walk faster, you have to get the signals to your muscles to fire faster. Sounds simple, but it takes some real physical effort and mental concentration.

To get beyond the 13-minute-mile wall, I taught a variation of interval training that runners use to increase their speed. Interval training involves fast work in short segments followed by recovery periods. For instance, a runner who competes in a mile race might run a quarter-mile interval at a faster pace than he could run the whole mile. He then slows down to a slow jog or walk for about a quarter mile to let his body recover before running a fast quarter again. A well-trained runner might repeat that cycle four to eight times in one workout session.

If you want to try a modified interval-training process, find a measured distance, like a high school quarter-mile track. Warm up for a mile, then blast off and try to walk a quarter mile in 3 minutes or less; that is the equivalent of a 12-minute-mile pace. Walk a slow, comfortable recovery quarter, then do another fast quarter. Repeat until you have done four fast quarters. Add up the times for the fast quarters, and you'll probably have a *total* time that is faster than a 13-minute mile.

By walking short, fast spurts, you are actually programming your brain to increase the firing of your walking muscles at speeds to which they are unaccustomed. It then becomes a matter of lengthening the process. I suggest that you do only four fast and four slow sessions (alternate them) per workout and only one interval workout per week.

In the early stage of aerobic walking, concentration is almost as important as the physical ability to sustain a fast walking speed, beyond the 13-minute mile. You will find that your speed drops if your mind starts to wander. Later on, as you become an accomplished aerobic walker and your muscles know how to fire faster, you will not have to focus your mind on them nearly as much.

There is a beneficial side effect from training your walking muscles to fire at a high intensity. It makes all your daily walking seem less enervating, and your normal walking pace will increase without any more effort. On a trip to EPCOT Center at Disney World several years ago, my wife, Carol, and I were comfortably walking along rubbernecking at all the sights when the couple we were with hollered for us to slow down. They were about 50 yards behind us. When I checked our speed, we were at the brisk pace, but it was as easy and comfortable as a stroll for us. All the aerobic walkers I know say the same thing—and so will you.

COULD IT BE SHIN SPLINTS?

The one thing I can predict with certainty that will happen as you accelerate your walk is *shin fatigue*. It generally hits most people somewhere between a 14- and a 13-minute-mile pace, but those who are quite a bit overweight may encounter it at slower speeds. Shin fatigue held me back when I first tried for the 12-minute mile, so don't be surprised or alarmed when it shows up on your walk.

Most walkers think they have shin splints, but they don't. Shin splints are generally a problem for runners. In *Conquering Athletic Injuries* (Leisure Press, 1988), Dr. David Bernstein explains, "Shin splints are caused by very small tears in the leg muscles at their points of attachment to the shin." He says they result from "muscular imbalances, insufficient shock absorption, toe running, or excessive pronation of the foot." These are running problems compounded by the foot's impact on the ground. I have yet to find an exercise-walker with a true case of shin splints.

It *is* common for exercise-walkers who are trying to move into the 12-minute-mile range to experience extreme fatiguing of the big muscle that runs down the front of the lower leg, along the shinbone. Its medical name is *tibialis anterior,* but we'll just call it the shin muscle. Although there are other muscles in the front of the lower leg, this is the one that is going to cause you some *temporary* discomfort.

In Figure 6.6 you can see the muscle I am talking about. It is often called the toe lifter because it is attached to the top of your foot and pulls your forefoot toward your shin so your foot will clear the ground as your leg swings under you. It also keeps your foot from flopping on the ground when you plant your heel and load your weight onto your foot.

Get to know and understand this muscle because, until you toughen it up, there will be times you will think it is on fire if you are walking faster than a 14-minute mile. You are already using this muscle in every step you take, but you are using it at a very low intensity. When you start walking at greater speeds, you use it at a higher repetition of work, and, like any of your other muscles, if it isn't conditioned for the workload, it will quickly fatigue, causing a burning sensation.

If you are seated, you can get a quick idea of how hard this muscle works. Pull your pant leg up to your knee and with your heel on the floor, but slightly in front of you, pull your forefoot slowly toward your shinbone as far as you can. You should be

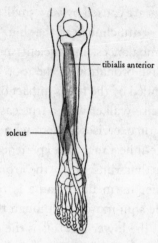

FIGURE 6.6

able to see the muscle bulge about 4 inches below your knee. Press your fingers on the muscle at the bulge and rock your foot up and down rapidly while keeping your heel on the floor. Do this quite a few times, and you will start to feel some fatigue even while sitting.

With your foot still slightly in front of you and your forefoot off the floor as if you had just planted your heel taking a step, rise out of your chair and load your weight onto that heel. Feel how hard the muscle is now. The shin muscle pulls your forefoot up on every step, and at heel plant it has to work to keep your forefoot from flopping to the floor as you load your entire body weight onto the foot. The muscle is actually stretched while it is actively developing contractile tension. According to Dr. Inman, it is "engaging in a lengthening contraction." In effect, it is working two ways at the same time.

In *Aerobic Walking,* I recommended some shin muscle exercises for conditioning, but, after several years of working with people in clinics, I have come to the belief that the best way to resolve shin muscle fatigue is to *walk it tough*. By that I mean walk at a speed that causes discomfort in the muscle, hold it as long as you can, then slow down to a pace where the discomfort disappears. Walk at that pace for about half the distance you just walked when the shin was uncomfortable, then pick up the pace and fatigue the muscle again.

In exercise physiology, this is called progression and over-load. You ask the muscle to work a little harder and a little longer each time, with periods of relaxation in between. Over time the shin muscle will toughen up and be able to handle the increased speed. When you can go a full mile without shin fatigue, you'll have it whipped. You'll be able to go 3, 4, or 5 miles also. It took me about two and a half weeks to get mine in shape, but I was 56 years old. I know younger walkers who got their shin muscles toughened in a week or less. The heavier you are, the harder those shin muscles have to work, but so do the rest of your muscles. It takes an overweight person somewhat longer to get the shin muscles fit.

A FEW DOS AND DON'TS

Do keep your elbows as close to your body with the bent-arm swing as they are when your arm is fully extended and hanging at your side. Many people have a tendency to stick their elbows out when they bend their arms. But having the elbows out from the body changes the position of the upper arm at the shoulder. When you swing your arms from that position, they will go across your body and lose their effectiveness as counterbalances for your legs. I call that chicken-winging.

To compare the proper elbow position with the chicken-winging position, bend your dominant arm 90 degrees at the elbow. With your upper arm hanging loose at your side, slowly bring it back so your loosely formed fist is at your hip, then slowly bring it forward till it is out in front of you (see Figures 6.3 and 6.4). Let your arm rock slowly back and forth like that a few times. If you are totally relaxed, your elbow should be close to your body and your forearm should lightly brush your rib cage just above your waistband. Your arm should swing back and forth as if it were in a groove. That's the groove you want when you are in full stride and your arms are swinging vigorously.

Now elevate your elbow away from your body about the width of a cantaloupe so you can see the floor between your elbow and your rib cage. Slowly bring your hand back toward your hip, then forward. You will see that the hand comes across your center line of gravity and above the breast. It is automatically guided that way because, by elevating your elbow out from your body, you have changed the way the upper arm rotates from the shoulder joint. Move your arm back and forth slowly to observe the path it takes, then pump it faster a few times. You can see that if you were walking fast and chicken-winging you would be getting counterproductive lateral arm movement. Keep those elbows close to the body; don't be a chicken-winger.

Do keep your shoulders in a natural, relaxed position. There is a great tendency among early students of the bent-arm swing to tense the upper body around the shoulders. I used to see it in all of my clinics, and I also had that problem in the beginning. Relax, relax, relax.

Don't hunch your shoulders as you increase your walking speed. I also struggled with this for a couple of weeks when I was learning. There is a tendency to elevate the shoulders as you accelerate your speed. It seems as if the shoulders want to touch the earlobes. I call this the Frankenstein look, and men seem more prone to it than women. When you break into a jog, your shoulders seem to elevate just at that moment. A walker walking at the pace of a jog sometimes gets his shoulders in that position too. It may not be a problem with you, but if it is, the solution is to relax, relax, relax.

Don't walk wide. As you learned in the last chapter, placing the feet in a wide track causes upper-body sway. At slower walking speeds this is not critical; it can be accommodated up to the midrange of the brisk pace fairly well. As you move up through the 13-minute-mile pace, though, unnecessary upper-body sway becomes counterproductive to forward progression and will affect your ability to become a smooth, fast walker. A narrow track, of 4 inches or less (measured as the width between the heels at their medial or inside edges at heel plant), keeps upper-body sway to a minimum.

An interesting way to observe upper-body sway is to walk with the sun behind you so that it casts your shadow directly in front of you. Walk at a brisk pace with your feet purposely tracking very wide and watch the side-to-side sway of your shoulders and head (some people walk this way all the time). Continue walking as you slowly decrease the width of your track until your feet land in a very narrow track. Upper-body sway should hardly be noticeable now.

Don't toe off until your trailing leg is well behind your pelvis. When you see people walking with their heads bobbing up and down (I call them bouncers), they are probably pushing off with their trailing foot still too close to and possibly even partially under their body. Remember when you stood with your feet under you and rotated your ankles by pushing against the floor with your forefoot, your body rose straight up. The lifting and falling action of the walking gait is exaggerated on the lifting part of the step cycle by toeing off too soon.

Although premature toe-off is not in any way injurious, it is biomechanically counterproductive and delays forward progression. It will also affect your ability to accelerate smoothly. In the stroll or brisk walk it is not a factor, but beyond a 14-minute mile it is. A narrow-track walker with the proper toe-off will be smooth and fast. A wide-track bouncer trying to walk fast will oscillate like an out-of-balance wheel on an automobile. I hate to keep harping on the gender differences between good walkers and bad, but I see twice as many wide-track men bouncers as women.

IT ISN'T RACE-WALKING

I originally felt that the complete race-walking technique was necessary to reach the aerobic range of walking. My clinical experience and that of the walking study at the Institute for Aerobics Research have since convinced me that the bent-arm swing coupled with your normal stride is all you need. Aerobic walking only has the bent-arm swing in common with race-walking. Put that together with correct posture and your normal stride, and you are on your way.

When walkers develop a good, coordinated aerobic walking technique, they really look smooth. Some women become so smooth and rhythmic in their walks that they actually look *sensual*. Look around the streets, parks, and shopping malls, and you will see more and more aerobic walkers using the bent-arm-swing technique every day.

AEROBIC WALKING CHECKLIST

We have covered all the biomechanical aspects of aerobic walking and how your walking gait must be managed to move up to the high-intensity level. I have thrown a lot of information at you, so here is a checklist to help you remember the key points.

- *Posture.* Posture is very important in the stroll and brisk paces but absolutely critical at the aerobic pace. Fatigue will set in quickly, especially in the shoulders and lower back, without proper posture. Chin up, head level, shoulders relaxed, hips in line under the shoulders, back straight, body erect. Do not compromise any of the foregoing in the interest of speed. Keep checking to make sure that your head is level and your chin is up and parallel to the ground. It is almost impossible for the shoulders to sag if your head is in the proper position. Scan the terrain ahead by lowering your eyes, not your head.
- *Arms bent 90 degrees at the elbow.* Hold your forearms up at a constant 90-degree angle at the elbows, and swing the arms from the shoulders with power and vigor in sync with your leg stride.
- *Arm swing.* Your forward arm swing should end with the hand slightly in front of your body (not across the center line of gravity) and no higher than the top of your breast. The back swing should go back till your loose fist is at your midbuttocks or behind the side seam of your shorts. Elbows and forearms should be close to your rib cage when they pass. Avoid chicken-winging. *Complete vigorous movement of the arms through the full swing cycle is extremely important.* Make sure your subdominant arm is

swinging with the same coordination and vigor as your dominant arm.

- *Hands.* Form a loose fist with the thumb resting on the first joint of the forefinger. Do not clench your fist and put tension in the arm muscles. Keep your hands and wrists in straight lines with your forearms.

- *Narrow track.* Try to walk a narrow track, about 4 inches or less measured from the inside edge of each heel at the point of heel plant. Avoid upper-body sway caused by wide-track walking.

- *Foot placement.* As the heel of the lead foot is placed on the ground, the toes should be up at a comfortable angle and pointing straight ahead. The forefoot should be lowered to the ground in a smooth, even manner with a *slight* emphasis on the outside edge of the foot. Avoid slapping the foot straight down from heel to toes.

- *Straight leg.* At heel plant, have your lead leg straight at the knee and keep it that way all the way through its weight-bearing phase as it passes under your body. Walking with high knee action is not smooth and often leads to placing the foot flat on the ground instead of with the toes up.

- *Toe-off.* The power of the step comes from the toe-off action of the foot. Make sure your trailing leg is well behind you so that your toe-off does not cause unnecessary rise of your body, creating a bouncy gait.

- *Shoulders.* Your shoulders should be squared to your line of travel and hang relaxed. The shoulder of the arm swinging forward will tend to rotate slightly forward with it. Do not try to increase this rotation. Let your shoulders function in a natural, relaxed manner.

- *Hip movement.* The hip has a slight natural rotation forward with the leg swinging forward. This movement varies greatly among individuals but seems more accentuated in women than in men. Walk with your hips under your shoulders and squared to your line of travel. Let them rotate in a natural, comfortable manner. You will notice more rotation as you increase speed.

- *Don't be Frankenstein.* Avoid hunching your shoulders as you try to walk faster. Doing so tenses your upper body and causes fatigue. It also distorts your posture and ruins your rhythm. Keep the shoulders down in their natural position and relaxed at all times.
- *Don't be Groucho Marx either.* Avoid the Groucho Marx creep by keeping your lead leg straight from heel plant to toe-off. A fast walk with bent knees ultimately converts to a flat-footed jog, in which you are using elastic energy instead of inefficient mechanical energy.
- *Putting it all together.* In order of importance, concentrate on posture, technique, rhythm, and speed. When all of these become one synchronized, fluid move, when you have perfect posture and are totally relaxed, when the ground flows by under your feet as you are smoothly cruising along—*then* you've got it all together.

Whether you exercise by the minute or the mile, there is no other aerobic exercise that is always as accessible, injury-free, and effective as aerobic walking.

FREQUENCY AND DURATION ARE MORE IMPORTANT THAN PACE

Even though I have introduced you to strolling, brisk walking, and aerobic walking, it is important to restate that *frequency and duration of exercise are more important than intensity for the general population.* Aerobic walking and possibly even brisk walking should only be attempted after you have established that you can walk about 3 miles per exercise session at least five times a week. Remember, the walkers in the study in Chapter 4 were all under 40 years old and they were able to adapt to the two faster paces because of their youth.

The first wave of baby boomers is turning 60 in 2006, with more on the way. Many of them are already experiencing health and weight problems that preclude their ability to accelerate their walk to the 15- or 12-minute-per-mile pace. The further up the age spectrum you get, the less pace is important or maybe even possible. In my late sixties I could still crank out 5 miles under 60 minutes, but now at 79 and with two artificial knees, I am all out walking 3 miles in 39 minutes. Most people my age (or even a lot younger) can't walk that fast, nor do they need to. I walk for a high level of fitness as well as my health, but between the two, health is more important.

If everyone (young, middle-aged, and old) would get up off their rusty, dusty rear ends and go out each day for a long walk, at whatever pace they can do *consistently,* we would see the nation's health soar and medical bills plummet. For many, good health is just a daily walk away.

SEVEN

Walking for Weight Loss and Weight Maintenance

I suspect that the majority of the people reading this book are involved in either a weight loss effort or a weight maintenance program. I am one of the latter. I guess I have gained and lost several hundred pounds over the past forty years, and as previously mentioned, at one time I was 52 pounds heavier than I am today. At age 79 I weigh 180 pounds, exactly what I weighed at age 22.

Since I have put together the right combination of exercise-walking and a healthful diet, my weight hasn't fluctuated 5 pounds in nearly a quarter century. I have won my battle—finally. The successful solution to my weight problem, yours, and everybody else's boils down to two factors: exercise (the right kind with adequate frequency and duration and ultimately intensity) and a heart-healthy diet. It is a photo finish as to which is more important, but it is a matter of record that those who have managed their weight problem the longest invariably are exercisers. The importance of a healthy diet will be discussed in the next chapter, but first let's tackle the major stumbling block for almost everyone—exercise.

The many diets that have come and gone over the years have generally consisted of some food combination or form of denial that would supposedly produce a dramatic weight loss. The low-carb craze featured in the Atkins diet is just one example. The primary emphasis in all of these diets has been on what and how much you eat; lip service was given to exercise. A consistent exercise regimen should be established *before* you start any form of diet modification. In order of importance it should be exercise and diet, not diet and exercise.

I strongly recommend that you start your exercise-walking program at least forty-five days before you attempt the diet aspect of weight loss. If you are successful with a *consistent* exercise program, reaching your weight goal is a slam dunk. Even more important, once you reach that goal, you will be able to maintain your weight at that level permanently—as long as you continue to exercise. It is an unassailable fact that consistent exercise is the key to proper weight loss and long-term weight maintenance.

In a January 17, 2005, *Newsweek* article on better aging, Dr. Howard Lewine, a faculty member at Harvard Medical School, answered a reader's question about whether it was possible to get back to her normal weight at age 60, after being overweight for eight years. He told her that it isn't merely a dream to become fit and trim at her age: "I recommend exercise as your first priority. As exercise becomes a regular part of your daily routine, start cutting calories. This is not a diet—it is eating less each day until your caloric intake becomes less than your daily energy expenditure. Weight loss will follow."

The most highly visible example of the foregoing is Oprah Winfrey. In 1988, dressed in skinny jeans and a long-sleeved dark top, Oprah wheeled a wagon loaded with fat onto the set of her show to represent her 67-pound weight loss. In a January 1991 *People* magazine article about Oprah Winfrey regaining the pounds she'd lost on her highly publicized liquid diet, Dr. Keith Berndtson, a weight-management specialist at Rush–Presbyterian–St. Luke's Medical Center in Chicago, stated: "The rate of regain on any weight loss regimen—not just liquid food replacement—is a whopping 95 percent, unless paired with exercise." According to *People*, Oprah had stopped exercising regularly and had gone back to eating her favorite foods, which are high in fat.

Oprah made a comment in *People* that goes to the heart of the problem: "I didn't do whatever the maintenance program was. I thought I was cured." Unfortunately, there is no "cure" for a weight problem. The problem always remains; one can only work to control it, and such control must be maintained one day at a time for the rest of your life. And think about this: if you don't control it, the rest of your life may be a lot shorter than you wish.

Yesterday's control was a victory, today's control is a battle being fought, and tomorrow's control is a new battle facing you. The role of exercise in these battles cannot be overstated. Consistent exercisers, particularly exercise-walkers, develop resolve, discipline, and an uncommon ability to take command of their lifestyle and make the changes necessary to control their weight problem. Oprah didn't have a chance to succeed without exercise, and neither do you.

As a longtime admirer of Oprah Winfrey, I watch her show as often as possible. Over the years she has gotten her weight back to a sensible level and has maintained it. On November 14, 2005, Oprah celebrated the twentieth anniversary of her nationally syndicated show, and in a St. Joseph News story (November 17, 2005) she referred to her 1988 show as her "biggest, fattest mistake." Oprah recalled, "I had literally starved myself for four months—not a morsel of food—to get into that pair of size 10 Calvin Klein jeans."

The difference between the 1988 Oprah and the 2005 version is her commitment to exercise and a healthful diet. On her shows from time to time she has her trainer, Bob Greene, talk about exercise and features healthful food programs to encourage her many viewers to follow her example. The operative word here is *commitment*. The January 2005 *Mayo Clinic Health Letter*, in an article about weight loss, stated, "Maintaining weight loss requires making a lasting commitment." Without a firm commitment to exercise, neither you, me, nor Oprah Winfrey will succeed in controlling a weight problem. It is for this reason that an exercise regimen should be established before tinkering with your diet. I tried it the other way more times than I want to admit, and I always failed. How about you?

The amount of exercise that is beneficial for the heart may not be sufficient for consistent weight loss or weight maintenance. Exercising three times or four times a week is good for cardiovascular fitness, but for weight loss or weight maintenance it is necessary to exercise nearly every day. Exercise is more difficult to sustain than dieting because it takes time and physical effort. Dieting, on the other hand, is passive, and while it requires significant mental discipline, it does not require physical exertion or the interruption of daily activities. For instance, you can be dieting while reading this book or watching a movie.

UNDERSTANDING FAT

There is no need to rush headlong into an exercise or diet program in an effort to lose fat unless you first understand its role in your physiological makeup. You don't cure excess fat, you control it, and what works sensationally for one person may be only moderately successful for another. In most cases the threshold of expectation about getting rid of excess fat exceeds the realities of how it can be done. Impatience is the biggest enemy of those in a weight loss program. Most don't really understand how their fat is accumulated and stored, or how it must be broken down chemically and used by the body as fuel to be eliminated.

Fat plays an important role in how our bodies function; it is only *excess* fat that creates problems. The textbook *Exercise Physiology* points out that the most noteworthy functions of body fat include providing the body's largest store of potential energy, serving as a cushion for the protection of vital organs, and providing insulation from the thermal stress of cold. It is the first that raises havoc with our weight. Most overweight people are simply storing more energy every day than they are using. Becoming overweight occurs when the *calories in exceed calories out*. The exceptions are those who have some specific medical reason for their excess weight, but they represent a very small percentage of the overweight population.

APPLES AND PEARS

If you are carrying excess body fat, are you shaped like an apple or a pear? The difference may determine your health risk and may influence whether it will be more difficult to get rid of your fat by exercise and dieting. Dr. Andrew Weil, clinical professor of internal medicine at the University of Arizona, in the June 2005 issue of his health letter *Self Healing,* addressed the differences in fat distribution between apple-shaped people and pear-shaped ones. He writes, "Not all kinds of body fat are created equal: it depends on where the fat is." Dr. Weil states, "People who are more likely to store excess weight in the abdomen have the so-called apple body shape, or what is known as central obesity. Those who deposit body fat primarily in their hips, thighs, and backsides are built like pears."

In an issue of *The Physician and Sportsmedicine* magazine (January 1991), Dr. Bryant Stamford discussed in detail the apple- and pear-shape fat accumulation: "Obese men tend to be shaped like apples, storing their fat above the waist, in the nape of the neck, shoulders, and abdomen. . . . Obese women on the other hand tend to be shaped like pears, storing their fat lower on the body, on the buttocks, and thighs." However, it can also go the other way, according to Dr. Stamford; men can be shaped like pears and women like apples.

The apples have good news and bad news. The good news is that they are able to reduce fat more easily than pears. The bad news is that the apple's fat poses increased heart attack risks and the propensity to develop diabetes. The excess dietary fat that is stored by apples is controlled by active enzymes. (The dictionary defines *enzymes* as "any of various proteins, as pepsins, originating from living cells and capable of producing certain chemical changes in organic substances by catalytic action, as in digestion.") According to Dr. Stamford, enzyme activity plays a role in calling fat from storage to be used as fuel.

Dr. Stamford stated: "Active enzymes may contribute to high cholesterol levels in apples because the greater amount of fat stored in the gut, the greater amount that can be dumped in the blood stream. . . . Enzyme activity increases when adrenaline is released during times of emotional stress and exercise stress causing fat stored in the abdominal cavity to be released into the blood stream."

This process is a mixed blessing. Exercising is good because it shunts blood flow toward the working muscles, fueling them with fat that you want to shed. But, as Dr. Stamford pointed out, during emotional stress this is bad, because fat-laden blood from the apple area is routed directly to the liver, providing it with abundant raw material for the production of artery-clogging cholesterol.

Additional bad news for apples is that abdominal fat cells tend to be larger than those in other areas of the body. Large fat cells are associated with glucose intolerance and an excess of insulin in the blood, which can develop into diabetes. In addition, according to Dr. Stamford, "excess insulin may promote reabsorption of sodium by the kidney, which may in turn lead to high blood pressure."

Metabolic problems such as high cholesterol and glucose intolerance increase the risk of coronary heart disease for apples. But nature seems to provide an escape hatch for some of the bad-news scenarios. Because the abdominal fat cells are so active and the turnover rate for abdominal fat is high, apples are able to reduce their abdominal fat more easily than pears are able to reduce fat on their hips, thighs, and buttocks.

There's more good news for apples. A study has shown that when fat is lost as a result of exercise, more is lost from the trunk area, where apples carry their weight, than from the extremities. Dr. Stamford said: "The message for apples is clear—get moving." I'll add that you can walk that gut off in less time than you think. You will not only look and feel better but also reduce your risk of heart attack, diabetes, and high blood pressure.

While pears don't face the same health risks that apples do, the fat they are carrying is more stubborn and harder to lose. Dr. Stamford referred to this fat as "gluteal-femoral pattern obesity." Research suggests that the reason fat is so stubborn on females is that the gluteal-femoral cells cling to their fat except during lactation. "This suggests that the female body zealously guards fat stores to ensure adequate energy support for nursing a baby," Dr. Stamford stated. Further studies have found that exercise training without calorie restriction reduces body fat in men but not in women.

Over and over in my walking clinics women asked, "Is walking good for reducing my hips and thighs?" Most women seem to be preoccupied with the size of their hips and thighs, but no exercise will spot-reduce a particular area of the body. The best any exercise can do is to help burn the body's excess fat, including that from hips and thighs. In this regard, exercise-walking works all of the major muscle groups in the lower legs, thighs, and buttocks. It can't get any better than that.

It seems that the deck is stacked against women who want to maintain their girlish figures. Childbirth brings on the most stubborn fat and puts it in the most obvious places. However, nature gives women an exercise advantage. I have repeatedly said that women are natural walkers, much better than men.

The combination of exercise-walking and a healthful diet will ultimately take fat off of hips, thighs, and everywhere else. I guarantee it!

UNLOADING EXCESS FAT

Filling the fat cells with more fuel than the body needs is generally a process of long-term, pleasurable overindulgence. Cheeseburgers, french fries, malted milk shakes, pizzas, cheesecake, and other heavy-fat foods did their job, and we loved every minute of it. Breaking all the excess fat down biochemically so that the body can use it as fuel is time-consuming and not always enjoyable or swift. Even if you are successful in getting it done by self-denial or some bizarre diet program, there is the specter of the 95 percent failure rate for keeping excess fat out of those cells for the rest of your life.

Exercise and altered diet composition, plus modest calorie restriction, are the surest ways to burn the excess fat that has accumulated in your fat cells. It is a slow process, but to be effective in the long term, it *should* be. Stop for a moment and estimate how long it took you to put all that excess fuel into your fat cells. Was it five, ten, or twenty years? In the lectures I conducted at the Cooper Wellness Program, I asked that question. The average age of the participants was 48, and it was a rarity that anyone in the group had put on all of his or her excess weight in five years or less; usually it had taken at least ten years.

The guidelines for the appropriate rate of weight loss are 1 to 2 pounds per week. An issue of the *Tufts University Health and Nutrition Letter* (January 1991) reported, "The slower the weight is taken off, the more likely it will be to stay off." There are two factors at work. First, you should not jolt your metabolic system with extreme calorie restrictions. Losing slowly is the healthy way. Second, and equally important, a permanent weight loss must be accompanied by a changed lifestyle that includes regular exercise and moderately reduced calorie intake. Lifestyles are not changed quickly. If you have the patience and determination to lose weight slowly while adapting to a new lifestyle, by the time you reach your weight goal, everything will be in place for it to become your permanent weight.

MATHEMATICS OF LOSING WEIGHT

One pound of body fat equals 3,500 calories. This means that if you are 25 pounds overweight, through the combination of exercise and calorie restriction you have to somehow create a deficit of 87,500 calories ($25 \times 3,500 = 87,500$) from your normal calorie intake. This number may seem enormous and unattainable, but think how many people try to do it by diet alone, without exercise. That is *really* doing it the hard way.

Creating a calorie shortfall of 87,500 by exercise and dieting is actually a very doable project. A realistic, easily attainable, weekly 1-pound weight loss goal would be to split the needed shortfall equally ($3,500 \div 2 = 1,750$) between extra calorie expenditure (exercise) and calorie reduction (diet). Thus, in an effort to lose 25 pounds at a rate of approximately 1 pound a week, you only need to exercise away 1,750 calories a week. You now need to reduce your calorie intake by a relatively small 250 calories a day ($250 \times 7 = 1,750$), which is the other half of your weekly goal.

Spinning off 1,750 calories per week with exercise-walking is going to take about 5 hours once you reach your frequency and duration goal (being able to walk an hour at a stroll, at least five days a week). By increasing your walking intensity to the brisk pace you will be burning approximately 350 to 400 calories per hour ($5 \times 350 = 1,750$).

There are 168 hours in each week. Anyone truly committed to long-term weight loss will find 5 hours out of the 168 for exercise. Two of the five hours can be done in two days (Saturday and Sunday) for an hour a day. This means that the other three hours could be done in the remaining five days at less than 40 minutes per day.

Those who are more aggressive and have the time can double the exercise for more weight loss and quicker results. Do not try to reduce your calories by more than 500 per day because that will put you in a caloric denial diet mode and, in the long term, you will most likely fail. However, do as much exercise-walking as you can *consistently*.

This neat mathematical equation of weight loss will not work with exact precision for everyone, but it is a realistic approximation. You might be pleasantly surprised to find that you lose more than a pound a week if you are an apple, or you may be a bit disappointed if you lose less, especially if you have the stubborn fat of a pear. Don't be impatient and raise your expectations too high. Even if it takes thirty weeks instead of twenty-five to reach your goal, that is only about seven months. I'll bet you didn't put on those 25 pounds in seven months—so why expect to take them off any sooner?

For most people, a lifetime exercise program is a major stumbling block. "I don't have the time" is the excuse used most frequently. In a country where the average family spends more than seven hours a day watching television (which contributes to the problem of obesity), this has a hollow ring to it. I have found that busy, motivated people who are truly committed to permanent weight loss and a permanent lifestyle change, almost without exception, find a way to get their necessary amount of exercise. Conversely, those who have more time but are not deeply motivated or convinced that exercise is part of the solution will always cite a lack of time.

There are also a great number of nonexercisers who use the lack-of-time excuse because they don't like any of the recommended exercises. That makes sense. None of us is going to do something that we don't like for very long, particularly a time-consuming activity. For this reason, exercise-walking has the greatest adherence and lowest dropout rates. Being natural, injury-free, and enjoyable should make it the exercise of choice for anyone attempting to lose weight and keep it off permanently.

Exercise Physiology states: "Evidence is accumulating to support the contention that exercise may be more effective than dieting for long-term weight control." The textbook indicates that it is becoming increasingly clear that people who maintain a physically active lifestyle or who become involved in endurance exercise programs maintain a desirable level of body composition. "Within this framework, a strong case can be made for habitual, vigorous physical activity for individuals of all ages."

LOSING FAT, GAINING MUSCLE, AND BURNING CALORIES

The use of exercise in a weight-loss program has a two-pronged favorable effect. In addition to burning excess fat, exercise helps the body develop lean muscle tissue. It helps you alter your body's composition away from a high percentage of fat, which encourages more fat storage, to a leaner, higher ratio of muscle to body weight. And muscle tissue burns more calories than fat does. Your weight-loss objective should be not just to lose weight but to lose fat and gain muscle.

Exercise Physiology says: "When considering exercise for weight control, factors such as frequency, intensity, and duration as well as the specific form of exercise, must be considered." It points out that continuous, big-muscle, aerobic activities that have a moderate to high caloric cost are the best. According to the textbook, "total energy expended" is the most important factor in the effectiveness of an exercise program for weight control.

The energy cost of a weight-bearing exercise such as exercise-walking is proportional to body weight. For instance, a 225-pound person will burn more calories than a 150-pound person when both are walking the same distance at the same pace.

The importance of burning 300 calories per exercise session is stressed in *Exercise Physiology:* "Although it is difficult to speculate precisely, as to a threshold energy expenditure for weight reduction and fat, *it is generally recommended that the calorie burning effect of each exercise session should be at least 300 calories* [emphasis in original]. . . . This can be achieved with 20 to 30 minutes of moderate-to-vigorous running, swimming, or bicycling or walking for 40 to 60 minutes." Exercise programs of lower caloric cost usually show little or no effect on body weight or body composition, according to *Exercise Physiology.*

As has been pointed out repeatedly, the exercise community continually downgrades walking as a vigorous or intensive exercise. *Exercise Physiology* has just done it again by advising that you can burn 300 calories in 20 to 30 minutes with moderate to vigorous running, swimming, or bicycling, but that it takes 40 to 60 minutes to do the same with walking. An important criterion has been omitted in this comment: the intensity of the walker. This has a significant effect on caloric expenditure.

Figure 7.1 displays research results from five countries on the energy expenditure of men who walked at speeds ranging from less than 1.0 mile per hour (slower than 60 minutes per mile) to 6.2 miles per hour (faster than a 10-minute mile). The different symbols in the chart represent the averages from the various studies, and I added the dotted lines to make it easy for you to see where calories burned per minute intersects with the speed of the walker. This intersection is extremely important because it clearly shows that walking intensity affects calories burned per minute of walking. Between a 20-minute mile (3 mph) and a 15-minute mile, there is only a 1-calorie-per-minute difference in energy expenditure. But beyond the brisk pace of 15-minute miles (4 mph), walking intensity has a dramatic effect. Increasing the walker's speed just 1 more mile per hour (the aerobic high-intensity pace of a 12-minute mile) almost doubled the calories burned per minute in this study.

Exercise Physiology states: "At faster speeds walking becomes less efficient and the relationship curves in an upward direction that indicates a greater caloric cost per unit of distance traveled." You bet it does! Once you move beyond the brisk 15-minute mile, you are in extended-gait territory, where the walking gait becomes highly inefficient. The increased walking intensity in Figure 7.1 of only 1 mile per hour, from 4 to 5 miles per hour, shows what a dramatic increase in calories burned per minute can occur when walking intensity is increased beyond a 15-minute mile.

Let's assume that three people of equal weight walked a dis-

FIGURE 7.1
ENERGY EXPENDITURE WALKING ON THE LEVEL AT DIFFERENT SPEEDS
Different symbols represent the mean values from various studies reported in the literature

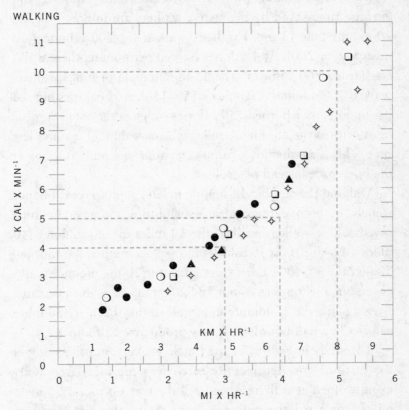

Source: W.D. McArdle, F.I. Katch, and V.L. Katch, Exercise Physiology: Energy, Nutrition, and Human Performance. *Philadelphia: Lee & Febiger, 1986.*

tance of 10 miles. As in Figure 7.1, their speeds varied: one person walked at 3 mph, another at 4 mph, and the third at 5 mph. Which one burned the most calories? Obviously the fastest walker burned the most calories by a substantial margin, and did it in considerably less time. With exercise-walking you can reduce your exercise time and increase your caloric expenditure simply by increasing your walking speed.

The actual numbers on the extra caloric expenditure and exercise time saved by the fastest walkers are impressive. The 20-minute-mile (3 mph) walkers walked for 200 minutes (10 miles × 20 = 200). At 4 calories burned per minute, these walkers burned 800 calories. The 15-minute-mile (4 mph) walkers walked 150 minutes (10 miles × 15 = 150). At 5 calories burned per minute, they burned 750 calories—almost the same number of calories as the 20-minute-mile walkers, but in 50 minutes less time. This is a reduction of almost an hour by simply walking at the brisk pace instead of strolling.

Walking the aerobic 12-minute mile (5 mph) pays off handsomely in both extra caloric expenditure *and* exercise time saved. These walkers walked the 10 miles in 120 minutes (10 miles × 12 = 120). At 10 calories burned per minute, they burned 1,200 calories, 400 calories *more* than the 20-minute-mile walkers and in a whopping 1 hour and 20 minutes less exercise time. Even against the 15-minute-mile walker, they burned 450 more calories in a half hour less. A very productive half hour!

The study in Figure 7.1 used male walkers, but the study at the Institute for Aerobics Research was the first large study using women at walking speeds all the way up to a 12-minute mile. I reported the percentages of their caloric expenditure based on walking speed in Chapter 4. In Figure 7.2, you can see how the results look on a chart prepared by Dr. John Duncan. Proving that gait efficiency is not gender-related, these women's caloric expenditures mirrored those of the men in Figure 7.1. The calorie-expenditure-per-minute scale shows that the aerobic 12-minute-milers burned more than twice as many calories per minute walking as the 20-minute-mile strollers did.

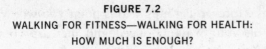

FIGURE 7.2
WALKING FOR FITNESS—WALKING FOR HEALTH:
HOW MUCH IS ENOUGH?

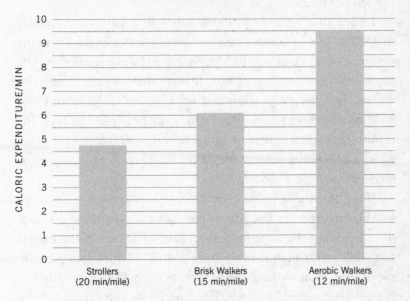

Source: Brown Shoe Co. Walking Study, Institute for Aerobics Research, Dallas, Texas.

In sum, walking speed is unquestionably related to energy expenditure for both males and females.

The same speed and duration may not be as effective when you near your weight loss goal as it was when you started. For example, if you are trying to lose 40 pounds, you will probably have to increase your walking duration and/or speed after you have lost 10 or 15 pounds in order to maintain the same rate of calorie burn per minute. That is a welcome challenge, however, if you are getting close to your weight goal. In a big weight loss program, the last 10 or 15 pounds are always the toughest and seem to take forever. Perhaps at this point you will want to really turn on your walking speed and increase your calories burned per minute.

I hope that exercise professionals will eventually recognize that walking a 12-minute mile burns more calories than walking slower. Some, however, will probably argue that most people can't and won't walk that fast. If reputable sources of exercise information keep repeating that walking isn't intense and that walking faster isn't important, why would people ever try? The caloric-expenditure benefit of increased walking intensity beyond a 15-minute mile is one of the best-kept secrets in the exercise field.

If the exercising public ever finds out about walking's intensity benefits for aerobic fitness and caloric expenditure, everyone, including the experts, will be amazed at how many people can walk faster than they thought possible. I am a living example of that. I am writing this chapter in early December 2005. It is a cold but sunny 28-degree day, and I have just returned from my 3-mile walk over a level country road. I walked it in 39 minutes flat—13 minutes per mile. I don't walk that fast every day. Tomorrow it might take me 41 minutes to walk the same course. I walk at the speed I feel like each day. Even so, I usually do it faster than 14-minute miles. I am not a race-walker; I walk for weight control and cardiovascular fitness. But because I know I can burn more calories in less time by walking fast, I do it and enjoy it, even at my advanced age. Ten years ago, I routinely walked this same course in 36 minutes or less. Father Time and a second artificial knee are the main factors in my slower times. Now that you know that walking speed really pays off by burning extra calories and reducing exercise time, maybe you will want to try to walk faster also. Physical exercise is exactly like mental exercise: you get out of it what you put into it.

When comparing walking intensity's caloric expenditure to other exercises that supposedly will burn more calories in less time, you will find that those exercises must be done at a vigorous rate far more challenging than walking a 14-minute mile or faster. Besides, what exercise can you expect to do vigorously four to seven days a week for a lifetime *except* walking? Add in the specificity principle, and you will wonder how any other exercise for weight loss could be recommended over walking.

THE WEIGHT LOSS PLATEAU

You are walking six days a week and eating a healthful diet with only moderate calorie restriction. The weight is coming off slowly and you are pleased with your program. But after about 20 or 30 pounds, the weight loss abruptly stops, even though you continue to do all the right things. This is the moment of truth called the weight loss plateau. It reminds me of the "stitch in the side" phenomenon, because it doesn't happen to everybody, and why it happens is not easily explained.

Unfortunately, if it lasts too long, a weight loss plateau causes a great number of people to throw in the towel. Usually they end up saying, "Exercise doesn't work." (For some reason exercise seems to get blamed more than diet.) In an issue of Weight Watchers' *Women's Health and Fitness News* (September 1990) Dr. Reva Frankle wrote: "Although the physiological causes of plateaus have not been fully studied the phenomena is a protective mechanism. . . . Faced with an ongoing caloric deficit that it interprets as starvation rather than safe dieting, the body puts on its brakes—and weight loss stops." For many this

brings about a crisis of confidence and, all too often, a weakening of will, because plateaus can last weeks, months, and even
up to a year.

The story of Dianne Anderson, a young music teacher from
Forest Park, Georgia, is the most extraordinary example of
willpower on a weight-loss plateau that I have ever encountered.
Dianne's experience was told in the October 1990 issue of *Prevention* magazine, and it will give you an idea of how tenacious
a weight loss plateau can be.

Dianne started at 321 pounds, with blood pressure that was
out of sight. Over three and a half years she lost 184 pounds; her
final weight was 137, and her blood pressure was now normal.
She did it by a combination of exercise-walking and a low-fat
diet. After numerous failed attempts on her own, she and a
friend started attending Weight Watchers. She received the counseling she needed for slow weight loss on a nutritional low-fat
diet. The accountability of weighing in each week added to her
commitment.

When she had lost 50 pounds by dieting alone, Dianne realized that she had so much more to lose that she would have to
exercise, so she started exercise-walking with the encouragement
of her friend. Unless you are extremely disciplined, exercise-
walking with a friend or a spouse is almost a prerequisite. Try to
hook up with another overweight walker for peer support.

In the first year, Dianne lost exactly 100 pounds, which
brought her down to 221. Then came the dreaded weight loss
plateau, and in the next year she lost only 30 pounds. At one
point she went four months without losing a pound. Dianne
said, "I knew what I wanted to do, and that my body was having to make adjustments. I clung to the fact that I wasn't going
to stop eating the healthy way I was eating whether I lost weight

or not. I was committed to eating that way for the rest of my life."

Dianne's walking was critical in bringing her through this crisis. It had given her confidence in herself that she had not had before. When she started walking, she weighed 270 pounds and walked for an hour at a time at whatever pace she could manage. She generally was able to go about 3 miles. "But," she said, "gradually I started going faster, till I could get in 4 miles. Then I didn't worry about trying to walk any farther; I just started walking faster."

On June 26, 1991, while researching the first edition of *Walking*, I spoke with Dianne, who had moved to Tempe, Arizona. She said that she still walked 4 miles a day, five days a week, for her weight maintenance of 137 pounds. She usually covered the distance in about 48 minutes, an average pace of 12 minutes per mile. From a snail's-pace beginning she was now burning up the roads—and the calories. Her combination of desire and discipline to conquer that four-month weight loss plateau is truly remarkable. I was unable to locate Dianne for this update, but based on the determination in her voice when I last talked to her, my guess is that she is still hanging tough with her walking and her weight maintenance.

MAINTAINING WEIGHT LOSS: THE TOUGHEST CHALLENGE

For many, getting the weight off is less of a challenge than keeping it off. Dianne Anderson took three and a half years to lose 184 pounds, and one whole year was a heartbreaker. Yet the ability to ride out delays and setbacks in a weight-loss program galvanizes individual resolve. Weight maintenance is a mindset that must take over after the biological battle to lose the weight has been won. In an issue of *Women's Health and Fitness News* (October 1990), Carol Morton, senior program developer at Weight Watchers, said: "Weight maintenance is a decision that has to be made early in a weight-control program—consciously and with commitment. . . . It goes beyond the dieting mentality, where the focus is on losing. In fact, reaching one's goal weight is really the beginning, not the end."

As pointed out earlier, exercise of any kind requires a time commitment and physical effort, whereas dieting does not. For those who don't have a full grasp of the importance of exercise, there is often a tendency to shorten it with a mental note to make up the needed caloric deficiency by dieting a little harder that day. Unfortunately, those kind of shortcuts tend to perpetuate themselves and exercise is ultimately abandoned. Long-term weight loss success is doomed when that happens.

Weight maintenance is most difficult for career women who are also raising families. In my walking clinics they told me that the demands of meals, laundry, dishes, cleaning, kids, and husbands (who, some said, are often more trouble than the kids), coupled with a full-time job, made finding time for exercise nearly impossible. Yet where there's a will there's a way. At an evening clinic I held in Houston years ago, I met Terri, a 33-year-old mother of two who worked full time as a paralegal. She was convinced that without her walking program she would gain back the 28 pounds she worked so hard to lose after the birth of her second child. This was exactly what happened to her after the birth of her first child, when she tried to keep her weight off with diet alone.

Terri was organized and committed, and she made sure that she got in 2 hours of walking every Saturday and Sunday. Three days a week she was at the nearby shopping mall when the doors opened at 6 a.m. She walked 45 minutes at a fast pace, then returned home before seven to get herself and her family off for the day.

Although Terri's schedule may seem exhausting, she said the walking actually elevated her energy level. After her first baby was born, when she didn't exercise, she was always logy and tired. Elevated energy level is common to all exercise-walkers, and it becomes an important contribution to weight maintenance. With a mind-set and a game plan, Terri was in control of her weight. As I bade her good-bye at the end of my clinic, she said, "I have to confess that some days it isn't easy." Then she smiled and added, "But anything really worthwhile rarely is."

TO WEIGH OR NOT TO WEIGH

A number of experts in the weight loss field recommend that you weigh yourself only once a week. This is a judgment call based mostly on the fact that your fat weight doesn't actually change much on a daily basis but your water weight may. If you happen to eat some highly salted food, for instance, you may show a gain of a pound or two overnight. The reasoning for weighing yourself only once a week is that a sudden one-day jump may cause you to get unwarrantedly discouraged.

I will give you the rationale why Carol and I weigh ourselves every day, and why we write our weight down on a scoreboard. First, however, it is important to have good scales. For a few dollars more than the little digital scales, some of which aren't very accurate, you can buy a doctor's-type scale with weights that slide back and forth on a bar. But whether digital or doctor's type, the scale should always be on a level, hard surface.

When weighing every day, it is important to weigh at exactly the same time, because your weight will fluctuate depending on food and liquid intake. Carol and I weigh ourselves when we get up every morning, before any intake of food or water. Our scale and clipboard with pencil are nearby. In the buff, we weigh ourselves and write our weight down next to the day's date. I never weigh myself at any other time of the day, and on those rare occasions when I am in a hurry and forget to do so in the morning, I don't bother until the next morning.

Weighing first thing in the morning and writing your weight down are helpful for two reasons. First, you get a consistent tracking of what your weight *really* is. Second, the fact that you know what it is at the start of each day means you have made a mental note of it. Your weight will keep coming back to haunt you like a bad check at every temptation you have to stray from your calorie counting or exercise plan.

Since my weight hasn't fluctuated 5 pounds in twenty-four years, why do I weigh myself every day? Perhaps that's why it hasn't fluctuated. I am always aware of my weight and I am also always aware of what my options are. Sometimes I eat something that I might not otherwise indulge in, like a couple of bites of a tempting dessert. And sometimes I have to say no thanks.

Another benefit of daily weighing is to familiarize yourself with your weight fluctuations. If you know why they occur, you won't push the panic button every time your weight jumps a pound or two. During the writing of this chapter, Carol and I went to dinner at our favorite Chinese restaurant. The next morning my weight was up a pound and a half. I shrugged it off because it always jumps like that when I eat at a Chinese restaurant. The extra weight is mostly water retention from the heavily salted food, not fat. In a day or two I am back to my regular weight. Knowing more about your weight fluctuations seems to me to be a much better way to control your weight after you have reached your goal. You will soon know whether the scale is weighing water or new fat. For instance, if your weight jumps a pound overnight, think back on what you ate and drank in the preceding 24 hours. Do a mental calculation to see if you actually consumed 3,500 more calories than you normally do. Unless you were involved in an unusual pig-out, which you would certainly remember, that extra pound is probably mostly water. The more you know about your body and how it functions, the better armed you are to make the right decisions about exercise and diet.

EXERCISE-WALKING AND CHILDHOOD OBESITY

The August 23, 2004, *Newsweek* cover story titled "When Fat Attacks" dealt in depth with our escalating national problem of obesity. In the same month *National Geographic* had a cover story titled "The Heavy Cost of Fat." It is not unusual for two major publications to address a national problem in the same month. However, the problem must be exceptionally wide in scope for a magazine such as *National Geographic* to stray from its normal topics to make it the cover story. And indeed it is.

Being overweight or obese was formerly generally considered an adult affliction, but as *National Geographic* pointed out, "Obesity has reached red alert levels among children and adolescents, almost tripling since 1980." For youngsters it is now at 15 percent and climbing. Childhood obesity was gaining momentum as far back as 1988, when *USA Today* in its July 25 issue ran a cover story about a 10-year-old girl trying to lose 52 pounds.

USA Today described in glowing terms how a fitness center

for kids in Virginia had structured a weight loss exercise program for this girl. The child had a serious weight problem and she had lost 12 pounds, according to the article, but still had 40 more to lose. "So the bright 10-year-old, a veteran of many failed diets, signed up for a special fitness program two months ago," the writer stated. A "veteran of many failed diets" at only 10 years of age? Sadly, she was about to become a failed exercise veteran as well, which at her tender age will undoubtedly turn her against exercise for many years, if not for life.

According to the article, the girl's exercise program to lose weight included "riding a stationary bike, weight training, using a rowing machine, jogging and playing games." By my count only one out of those five has any long-term merit as exercise for a 10-year-old girl or boy. Games are fun at 10 years of age, and, while they may not be aerobic, they will at least keep this girl active and interested. Exercise equipment is a quick burnout for most adults and probably has no chance at all with kids. According to *USA Today,* the child said, "I don't like running, but I have to do it for my program so I am starting to like it more." When a 10-year-old says, "I have to do it," she is simply saying that some adult has told her this is her medicine and she has to take it. When it comes to exercise, whether 10 or 60 years old, no one will do something they don't like for very long.

The heading of the story's continuation read "Make Sure It's Fun." Does anyone reading this think that what I have just told you would be "fun" if *you* were an overweight 10-year-old? By what stretch of the imagination could you envision that an exercise cycle, rowing machine, weight machine, and jogging would be fun for anyone at any age, let alone a 10-year-old? The most obvious flaw in this weight loss program was the total absence of exercise-walking. Those young legs and lungs are ideally suited for the bent-arm-swing aerobic walking. Hook an iPod on her with some of her favorite rock or rap music, and this young girl could burn a lot of calories every day while truly having fun. And when she is 40 there is a good chance that she will still be walking. It is doubtful that she'll be using an exercise cycle or a rowing machine and jogging.

I believe the family that walks together loses weight together. Chances are, if you have an overweight child (or children) you and/or your spouse probably have a weight problem also. If so, what better physical and mental support could you give your child than to help him or her (and yourself) lose weight with a family walking program? Take turns setting the pace, letting your child do it one day and you the next. Make it a fun and challenging experience to keep your youngster's interest. In the process, you will be both losing weight and bonding as a family. It is a win-win situation for everybody.

For an obese 10-year-old, or for an obese adult, the solution to weight loss and weight maintenance is the same. Consistent exercise is essential, and the important role that exercise-walking can play as the most sustainable, effective, injury-free exercise is undeniable. From time to time, I have been accused of being overzealous about exercise-walking, and, frankly, I am. What a wonderful thing to be overzealous about. Measured against all of the other exercises, it is in a class by itself.

A WALKING LIFESTYLE

Whether you are about to embark on a weight loss program or are struggling to maintain the weight you now have, exercise-walking at an intensity level that you can attain consistently should become as important to you as bathing or brushing your teeth. Embrace it as a welcome part of your daily lifestyle. You will enjoy walking, and you will enjoy even more the confidence of knowing that you have your weight problem under control *permanently*. It doesn't matter if you are as obese as Dianne Anderson was. Start walking as she did, slowly but consistently. And remember, walking is not a beginner's bridge to more-vigorous exercise; walking is a bridge to a happier, healthier life.

EIGHT

Eating Smart, Living Lean, and Living Longer

They that take medicine and neglect diet waste the skill of the physician. —Chinese proverb

There's an old saying that man is the only animal who eats when he is not hungry, drinks when he is not thirsty, and has sex in all seasons. One of the three isn't fattening—so enjoy! Exercise and its importance was covered in the previous chapter, but as I pointed out, it is only half of the weight-control equation. The other equally important half is diet—not diet as in denial but diet as in the composition of daily food intake. It was the combination of exercise and a low-fat, high-complex-carbohydrate, heart-healthy diet that enabled me to stabilize my weight exactly where I wanted it after years of losing and gaining, losing and gaining. That combination will also work for you.

The purpose of this chapter is to alert you to some of the dietary pitfalls facing every unknowing, unsuspecting, health- and weight-conscious person, and to show you how important it is to eat smart. Learning a few things, such as how many calories are in a gram of fat and how to read a food label, will help you immensely to eat healthy and thus control your weight—as long as you exercise. We can't forget that. We all tend to overestimate how much exercise or physical activity we do and underestimate how many calories we consume.

In my earlier years I was a sucker for every quack diet that came along in an effort to find a quick, easy solution to my weight problem. Trust me, there isn't one. If you accept the fact, as I did, that excess weight is a major risk factor to your health, then you will do what it takes to protect yourself. Getting the weight off and keeping it off requires more than just exercise and diet. It involves a strategy and a continuous effort.

FIVE THINGS SUCCESSFUL DIETERS DO

Some people successfully lose weight and keep it off, and many others fail. This is the dilemma the National Weight Registry has been looking into for over a decade. Since 1994, the registry has amassed information on nearly five thousand people who have maintained at least a 30-pound weight loss for five or more years. Periodically, they are interviewed to see what makes them able to stick to their goals. In the August 2005 *University of California, Berkeley Wellness Letter* they list the key strategies the successful maintainers use, according to Dr. James Hill, the registry's cofounder. The strategies include a diet high in complete carbohydrates such as fruit, vegetables, and high-fiber foods, and low in fat; being conscious of calories; eating breakfast; weighing yourself once a week; and doing 60 to 70 minutes of physical activity a day. The letter lists walking as their favorite suggested activity.

I had not heard of the National Weight Control Registry until I started research for this update, but everything in the foregoing list is exactly what I have been doing for the past twenty-four years—and my weight hasn't fluctuated five pounds in all of those years. Following these guidelines works for me, works for the people in the registry, and will work for you.

The *UC Berkeley Wellness Letter* listed some other critical information from the registry. It said, "Most people who become successful maintainers have failed several times before. Hardly anyone gets it right the first time around." I am living testimony to that, as I admitted earlier.

Failing is fairly normal, so don't feel you are a loser if you fail a few times. Take a long hard look in the mirror at the person looking back at you. If you see that you are truly overweight—particularly if you are obese—you must realize that you are in a grave danger zone for your health. Quality of life and expectations for a long life are greatly diminished. Pick yourself up and try again, and again, and again. Above all, don't give up! As an English proverb says, don't dig your grave with your own knife and fork.

The January 9, 2006, issue of *People* magazine devoted its cover story to ten men and women who lost from 100 to 300 pounds. Many cut their weight in half or more. The largest loss of weight was by a man, Rick Salewske, who went from 538 pounds down to 238. As *People* said, they did it "the old-fashioned way: cutting portions, taming cravings and working up a sweat." None did it with a surgical procedure.

The details of what they ate revealed that some opted for portion control plans such as Jenny Craig or NutriSystem while others controlled their own portions. Either way, to succeed they had to consider calories coming in and calories going out. The one thing they all had in common for calories going out was consistent exercise, and most started out walking. A few have converted to some running, but the majority are still walking. That is no surprise to me. Eight out of the ten people featured in the article were women, and I'll say it again: women are excellent natural walkers.

People also featured one of its weight loss cover girls from 2005, Dacia Gilkey, who lost 122 pounds and has kept it off. Ms. Gilkey said she keeps close tabs on her weight. If the scale shows she has gained a few pounds, that's her cue to step up her five hour-long weekly workouts. *People* says, "Gilkey complements her workouts with grilled chicken, vegetables, brown rice and salad." That sounds like she is on a low-fat, high-complex-carbohydrate diet, which is what I follow.

This chapter is meant not to give you a detailed menu for a specific weight-loss diet but to clue you in on where the dietary land mines are in a grocery store, and what are the healthful foods and reliable sources of information. Sadly, as a nation we are nutritionally illiterate. I used to include myself in that category. I was well past 50, a college graduate, and a successful businessman, but nutritionally I was dumber than a retarded ox. I used to order a double cheeseburger, a large order of fries, and a Diet Coke. See what I mean?

Only after I decided to seriously lose weight and keep it off did I start to study about what I was senselessly shoving down my gullet every day. It was then that I realized how little I knew about nutrition.

One of the first things everyone should know is that a gram of fat has nine calories and a gram of carbohydrates has only four calories. You've probably heard the old trick question, "What weighs more, a pound of lead or a pound of feathers?" It is not a trick question, however, when I ask, "Which one is larger?" Obviously, the density of lead makes it the smallest. Consider a similar comparison question, "Which takes up the most room, 500 calories of fat or 500 calories of complex carbohydrates?" The nine-to-four calorie ratio makes fat much denser. A small portion of food high in fat can pack a lot of calories per ounce, which makes it easier to eat more of it than you should. Not only are fruits, vegetables, and whole grains healthy foods, but their volume per calorie permit you to eat more and avoid hunger pangs.

The *Mayo Clinic Health Letter* explains the health aspects of weight control and the role of dietary fat in their June 2005 issue. It states, "Weight-loss diet fads come and go. Sometimes, official recommendations for a healthy diet also change. But no matter what you hear, limiting fat in your diet—particularly saturated fat and trans fat found in processed foods containing partially hydrogenated oils—is one of the most important dietary changes most Americans can make for optimum health."

The letter continues, "An overwhelming amount of evidence has shown that low-fat, plant-based diets emphasizing vegetables, fruits and whole grains are associated with dramatically lower risks of cancer and cardiovascular diseases such as heart attack and stroke." And here is their clincher: "In terms of weight loss—or avoiding weight gain—decreasing the amount of fat in your diet is the most effective way of reducing the amount of calories you consume. That's because 1 gram of fat has 9 calories and 1 gram of carbohydrate has only 4 calories."

Ounce for ounce, you get less than half the calories per serving of equal weight when you eat carbohydrate calories—preferably complex carbohydrates—instead of fat calories. All nutrition labels list fat, carbohydrates, and protein in grams. To establish the relationship of ounces and pounds to grams here is an easy guide to help you read nutrition labels:

1 pound (lb) = 454 grams (g)
1 ounce (oz) = 28 grams (g)
1 gram (g) = 1,000 milligrams (mg)
1 milligram (mg) = 1,000 micrograms (mcg)

On food labels, the key equivalence to remember is that 1 ounce = 28 grams. To get a perspective on relative weight, 1 gram is about what a paper clip weighs.

GOOD-BYE, DIET

Kathy Duran-Thal is the registered dietitian who teaches at Dr. Kenneth Cooper's Wellness Program in Dallas, Texas, where I taught exercise-walking for six years in the 1990s. She teaches participants everything they need to know about low-fat eating, low-fat cooking, how to shop for low-fat foods, and how to stock a low-fat kitchen. I have eaten many of her delicious lunches and dinners, which have less than 20 percent fat in them. She is the source for much of the information in this chapter.

Kathy greets her new wellness participants with these words: "It should comfort you to know that the best diet is no diet at all. Why? Because typically you go on a diet until you reach your goal and then you return to the 'normal' eating habit that got you in trouble in the first place. Also, many diets encourage imbalance by restricting or emphasizing a particular food group. This kind of diet is difficult to maintain and over time could become dangerous to your health. Whether you need to lose, gain or maintain: make health your priority."

Kathy further counsels the participants: "Experience has taught us that small changes sustained over a long period of time lead to permanent weight loss. Make gradual changes, changes that will remain with you throughout your life. As you lose fat and gain muscle you will look and feel great. Once you begin eating smart, good things follow: energy levels increase, excess pounds fall away, and weight control becomes easier. If your lifestyle doesn't control your diet then eventually your diet will control your lifestyle."

GOOD FAT AND BAD FAT

Not all fat is bad. A certain amount of fat is necessary to maintain optimal health. Fat supplies energy, contains essential fatty acids, and enhances the flavor and texture of food. On the other hand, excessive consumption of fat is linked to higher cholesterol levels, heart disease, diabetes, cancer, and obesity.

There are many types of fat; some are beneficial and some are not. No matter what type food they are in, fats are a mixture of three different fatty acids: monounsaturated, polyunsaturated, and saturated. The proportion of each type of fatty acid determines the physical characteristics of a fat and its effect on human health.

Monounsaturated fatty acids are liquid at room temperature.

Oils such as olive, peanut, almond, and canola are high in mono-unsaturated fatty acids, as are avocados, olives, peanuts, and almonds. These may help lower blood cholesterol levels when used instead of fats such as butter or stick margarine and are considered a "good fat."

Polyunsaturated fatty acids are liquid or soft at room temperature. They are found in foods such as seafood as well as corn, safflower, soybean, and sunflower oils. These oils may also help lower cholesterol and are considered a "good fat."

Saturated fatty acids come primarily from animal products as well as coconut, palm, and palm kernel oils. As a general rule, they are more solid at room temperature. Examples include butter, stick margarine, shortening, and the fat in cheese and meat. Saturated fats have the most impact on increasing blood cholesterol levels. This is considered a "bad fat."

Remember this: *While the first two fats are not considered harmful from a cholesterol standpoint, all three fats have nine calories per gram, and all three fats are equally fattening.* The typical American diet gets an average of between 40 and 50 percent of its calories from fat. The American Heart Association recommends that you limit saturated fat to 10 percent or less of your daily calories and reduce your total fat intake to 30 percent or less. There is some growing speculation that even 30 percent fat may be too much in the long term. Certainly reducing your total fat intake to 20 percent or less will help you reach your weight goal more quickly and more safely.

Trans fat is another "bad fat" that is on a par with saturated fat. In January 2006 the Food and Drug Administration (FDA) added trans fat to the nutrition label right under saturated fat. All foods with half a gram or more per serving must list the amount they contain. Research shows that trans fat has a negative effect on cholesterol. Trans fat is an artificially created type of fat. Unlike the other fats, trans fat does not occur naturally in foods but is created when hydrogen is added to liquid oils, which makes it resist going rancid and adds to the shelf life of the product. If you look at the ingredients list on a food package and see that some of the oils are hydrogenated or partially hydrogenated, you can bet the food has trans fat.

Trans fat shows up mostly in baked goods such as doughnuts, cookies, and cakes. Since the FDA began to require the listing of trans fat, many food processors are changing their recipes to reduce it or eliminate it. Unfortunately, however, restaurants and fast food outlets do not have to comply with the FDA requirement, and they can be a major source of trans fat. Be careful and don't order anything fried. For instance, a large order of french fries cooked in hydrogenated oils will have about 6 grams of trans fat. That is a lot of fat sludge to pump through your arteries.

Try to aim for zero trans fat in your diet because it has no positive nutritional benefit and contributes to heart disease. If a food processor is more concerned about its product's shelf life than your life, then let them leave it on the shelf. There are plenty of other healthful foods you can buy.

Omega-3 fatty acids are polyunsaturated fatty acids found primarily in seafood, especially higher-fat cold-water varieties such as salmon, tuna, mackerel, and lake trout. Omega-3 fatty acids are good for the heart and brain, and may even aid in the treatment of depression. This is a "good fat." Most heart-healthy diets recommend cutting back on meat to reduce saturated fat and increasing fish consumption. But remember, a calorie is still a calorie—don't go overboard.

Three of the most widely used and popular "good" oils are

olive oil, canola oil, and soybean oil. Each has its strong and weak points. The best kinds of fat found in oil are first, mono-unsaturated fat, and next, polysaturated fat. Saturated fat should be kept to a minimum. However, don't go overboard with any kind of oil.

Olive oil, which is part of the heart-healthy Mediterranean diet, is 78% monounsaturated fat and 9% polyunsaturated fat, which is very good. It is not commonly known, but olive oil has 14% saturated fat. Canola oil is probably the best of the "good" oils. It is composed of 62% monounsaturated fat, 31% poly-unsaturated fat, and only 7% saturated fat. Soybean oil, an in-expensive and wisely used vegetable cooking oil, has 24% monounsaturated fat, 61% polyunsaturated fat, and 15% satu-rated fat.

Remember that *all* fats (good and bad) have 9 calories per gram and are equally troublesome in terms of losing weight.

HIGH CARBS OR LOW CARBS?

The enthusiasm for the low-carb diet as touted by the late Dr. Robert Atkins has died down, but during its heyday it had a lot of people believing they had found the "magic bullet" for weight loss. I didn't go for it because I had already tried it a couple of decades earlier when his first book was published. It appealed to me because I dearly loved bacon, sausage, steak, eggs, and all of the fatty foods Atkins said you could eat. It sounded like meal-time nirvana. I was only able to stay with it a couple of weeks and all I got out of it was bad breath and constipation. It was another of the many failed magic diets that I tried.

The body processes fat calories and carbohydrate calories differently, and, according to Dr. Bryant Stamford in a May 1990 article in *The Physician and Sportsmedicine* magazine, the body easily converts dietary fat to body fat. This conversion process uses only 3 calories per 100 calories consumed, meaning that 97 fat calories out of 100 can be stored as body fat. And there's a wrinkle you may not be aware of. According to Dr. Stamford, "Fat storage is accelerated when you consume fat and simple sugar at the same meal—combining a sugared cola and french fries for example. . . . Sugar triggers the release of insulin and insulin activates fat cell enzymes which promote the passage of fat from the bloodstream into fat cells."

A shift to more intake of complex carbohydrates can reduce fat storage even when you don't reduce your calorie intake. According to Dr. Stamford, this is true for three reasons. The first is that carbohydrates can be stored as glycogen, which prevents their conversion to fat. Even though glycogen storage is limited, Dr. Stamford said, "the body can expand storage capacity in those who regularly consume large amounts of carbohydrates and in those who exercise regularly."

The second reason is that when maximum storage capacity is reached, the body increases its metabolic rate to burn off excess carbohydrates. Third, there's a bit of a safety valve when storage and increased metabolism are inadequate to handle the carbohydrate load and the body has to convert the excess to fat. Dr. Stamford pointed out that this conversion process is calorically costly; it requires 23 calories out of every 100 calories of carbohydrates consumed. This means that only 77 out of 100 calories would be stored as fat.

These three factors ensure that "less body fat results from carbohydrate calories than from an equal number of fat calories," Dr. Stamford wrote. "The bottom line: If optimal health and slender physique are your goals, a low-fat, high-carbohydrate diet coupled with mild, comfortable exercise will accomplish much more than vigorous exercise coupled with a high-fat diet."

Carbohydrates are either simple or complex and both are eventually converted to sugar. The way the body absorbs them determines whether you should eat a lot of them or just a few. Complex carbohydrates include such foods as fruits, vegetables, grains (whole-wheat flour, brown rice), beans, cereals, and soy products in their natural forms. These foods are rich in fiber, which slows their absorption. These are the kind of heart-healthy foods recommended by the American Heart Association.

In contrast, simple carbohydrates such as refined sugar, white flour, white rice, alcohol, and others are absorbed by the body quickly. This causes a rapid rise in blood sugar, promotes an insulin spike, and eventually accelerates the conversion of calories into triglycerides, which is how the body stores fat. Reducing these kind of carbohydrates makes sense, but substituting artery-clogging, high-saturated-fat foods for healthful foods that contain complex carbohydrates does not.

Complex carbohydrates are nature's gift to good nutrition—they are low in fat and calories, cholesterol-free, and rich in vitamins, minerals, and fiber. The Institute of Medicine's Food and Nutrition Board recommends that the majority of our daily calories (45–65 percent) should come from these plant-derived foods. With simple carbohydrates the rule of thumb is *moderation*. Satisfying your sweet tooth now and then can be part of a balanced diet if you don't go overboard. Your health goal is to make your life longer, not just make it seem longer.

If you want to go on a 1,500-calorie diet and want to know how many grams of fat equals 30 percent fat calories here is an example:

$$1,500 \text{ calories} \times 0.30 = 450 \text{ calories from fat}$$
$$450 \text{ calories} \div 9 = 50 \text{ grams of fat}$$

Reducing the diet to 20 percent fat calories would go like this:

$$1{,}500 \text{ calories} \times 0.20 = 300 \text{ calories from fat}$$
$$300 \text{ calories} \div 9 = 33.3 \text{ grams of fat}$$

Fat grams for other amounts of total caloric intake can be figured using the same formula.

THE TRICKY FOOD LABELS

If you plan to reduce your calories and fat intake, perhaps the biggest unexpected obstacle you may face will be some of the major food companies. They have found that rich, sweet, fat, oversalted food appeals to more taste buds than more healthful, less sweetened, low-fat, lower-sodium food. Obviously they are going to put on the grocery shelves what sells the best. You have to be able to sort out the overprocessed foods from the nutritious, healthful foods, and therefore you must learn how to read and fully understand nutrition and ingredient labels.

Kathy Duran-Thal says surveys reveal that Americans will spend up to 33 percent more for a product with the word *natural* on the label. Are you aware of the many other nutritional buzzwords that food processors print prominently on their brightly colored packages? For instance, suppose you saw an attractively colored box on the grocery store shelf with the following in big letters: "Low-calorie, low-fat, low-sodium, no cholesterol, no sugar added, no preservatives, no additives, no artificial coloring, high-fiber, and 100% natural." Sounds like the perfect health food, doesn't it? Be careful, it could also be a box of fresh horse manure. Don't get taken in by nutritional buzzwords.

The information you really need will probably be in smaller print near the bottom on the side or back of the package. This is usually where you find the nutrition label and/or ingredient labels, which contain information required by the Food and Drug Administration (FDA) and the U.S. Department of Agriculture (USDA), plus some information supplied at the option of the food processor. This is where you find the information you need to make a proper buying decision.

Under FDA regulations revised in 2006, the Nutrition Facts label tells you how many calories and how many grams of protein, carbohydrates, and fat (including trans fat) are in a serving of the product. The label also lists the percentages of the U.S. recommended daily allowances (U.S. RDAs) of protein and seven important vitamins and minerals in each serving. The label tells you the size of a serving (for example, 1 cup, 2 ounces, 1 tablespoon) and how many servings there are in the container. The ingredients may be listed with the nutrition facts or in another area of the package. Ingredients in the largest amount by weight must be listed first, followed in descending order by weight of the other ingredients.

Grocery store aisles are filled with caloric land mines. Tiptoeing through them to buy the right kinds of healthful foods is a nutritional game of wits. You must take the position that many food companies are more interested in your wallet than in your waistline. If it's in a box, bottle, jar, can, or package and doesn't have a complete nutritional food label on it revealing how many fat grams, cholesterol, and sodium are in it, I don't buy it—and neither should you. Always look for a product that is fully labeled so you can make a buying decision based on accurate nutritional information.

To get a comprehensive explanation of *all* the aspects of a nutrition label, go to the FDA's Center for Food and Applied Nutrition's excellent website, www.cfsan.FDA.gov. On the upper left of the home page is a box labeled "Select a topic." Scroll down to "Nutrition" and click "Go." When the "Information About Nutrition" page comes up, click on "How to Understand and Use the Nutrition Facts Label." It will tell you everything you need to know.

In the past decade, the emphasis on meat has swung from beef and pork to poultry as a healthier choice from the standpoint of cholesterol and saturated fat. Turkey breast without the skin is considered the lowest in cholesterol and saturated fat. This part of the turkey has only about 18 percent fat calories. You can buy packaged turkey breasts that are cooked and ready to eat, but what do they do with the rest of the turkey? They make ground turkey, turkey bologna, turkey salami, and turkey pastrami out of it. Judging from the fat numbers on those products, they must throw in everything, including the gobble.

I bought a lot of ground turkey and turkey bologna before I found out it wasn't as healthful to eat as turkey breast. For instance, a 4-ounce serving of Louis Rich ground turkey contains 11 grams of fat. It has 180 calories per serving, but 100 of those calories are from fat—over 50 percent! Oscar Mayer turkey bologna has 4 grams of fat and 50 calories per serving, of which 35 are fat calories—70 percent. By comparison, Oscar Mayer light beef bologna also has 4 grams of fat, 60 calories per serving, and 35 fat calories—almost the same as turkey bologna. A serving is only 1 slice, which weighs 1 ounce (28 grams). Add up the number of slices you think it would take to make a tasty sandwich and then multiply the calories and fat calories. See how easy it is to underestimate how many calories and how much fat you are eating?

As you begin to alter the composition of your daily diet to get its fat content down below 30 percent, you might as well forget sausage and processed lunch meats. Almost all of this kind of meat has more than double the percentage of fat you should be eating, which means you would have to cut back more severely on all of your other fat intake. If you can decrease your meat consumption and increase fruits and vegetables, you will be well on your way to mastering your fat and calorie intake, and well on your way to mastering your weight problem.

PORTIONS: EITHER TOO SMALL OR TOO BIG

In my view, the portion sizes used to calculate calories, cholesterol, and saturated fat content for unprocessed meat are too small and totally unrealistic. Those portions are 3 ounces. Where can you order a 3-ounce steak? The petite filet mignon (the smallest) is 6 ounces in every restaurant I have patronized. What supermarkets cut and package steaks in 4-ounce sizes (generally 4 ounces raw = 3 ounces cooked)?

I have read that the average portion of meat eaten per meal is about 5.4 ounces. Consequently, if you see a TV commercial for the beef industry touting only 150 calories per 3-ounce serving, you may as well double that number for the real world. The same goes for poultry and pork. All of the numbers quoted are about half of what a person eats at an average meal. On special occasions, it may be only a third. It is this kind of impractical information that causes people to eat more calories, cholesterol, and fat than they realize—and more than they should.

Figure 8.1 lists the calories, fat, saturated fat, and cholesterol in various cuts of beef, pork, and poultry. In this chart, too, the numbers given are for the unrealistic 3-ounce servings.

FIGURE 8.1
GOOD CHOICES FOR REDUCING FAT AND CHOLESTEROL

Name of cut	Calories	Fat (grams)	Saturated fat (grams)	Cholesterol (milligrams)
Beef (lean only, choice grade)				
Top round steak, broiled	165	5.49	1.92	72
Eye of round, roasted	156	5.68	2.17	59
Tip round, roasted	164	6.59	2.41	69
Sirloin, broiled	180	7.69	3.14	76
Top loin, broiled	176	7.99	3.20	65
Tenderloin, broiled	176	8.15	3.18	72
Bottom round, braised	191	8.47	3.01	81
Chuck arm pot roast, braised	199	8.77	3.33	85
Pork (lean only)				
Tenderloin, roasted	141	4.09	1.41	79
Ham, boneless, water added, extra lean (approximately 5% fat)	111	4.23	1.38	39
Ham, cured, center slice	165	7.08	2.37	not available
Center loin chop, broiled	196	8.91	3.07	83
Poultry (roasted)				
Turkey, light meat, without skin	131	2.48	.79	59
Chicken breast, meat only	140	3	.86	72
Chicken drumstick, meat only	146	4.8	1.26	79
Chicken breast, meat and skin	167	6.6	1.86	71
Chicken drumstick, meat and skin	184	9.47	2.59	77

Figures for 3-ounce cooked servings, with all visible fat removed and prepared with no added fat.

Source: U.S. Dept. of Agriculture Handbooks No. 8–5, 8–10, and 8–13.

Now that people are eating more poultry (chicken and turkey) to reduce cholesterol and saturated fat intake, they may be kidding themselves about fat intake if they don't eat the right piece and remove the skin. Check the bottom number in the fat column: 9.47 grams of fat for 3 ounces of chicken drumstick meat with the skin. Now check the other numbers in that column; that piece of chicken has *more* fat grams than any of the lean beef or pork. Notice also that a chicken breast with skin has more than double the fat grams of one without skin.

Choosing the right meat and watching the portion sizes are a good start. Kathy Duran-Thal advises avoiding heavily marbled or fatty cuts—for example, corned beef, bacon, pastrami, spareribs, short ribs, rib eye roast or steak, most ground meats, frankfurters, sausages, most lunch meats, goose, domestic duck, and organ meats, such as liver and sweetbreads. Organ meats are also the highest in cholesterol.

Duran-Thal says the best choices to reduce fat as a percentage of total calories and cholesterol are fish and shellfish (but you should limit shrimp because of its high cholesterol content to no more than a couple of servings per week), along with chicken and turkey (particularly the white meat with all skin removed), lean beef, veal, pork, and lamb, trimmed of all visible fat. Limit red meat to a maximum of two or three servings per week, and have no more than 6 ounces of meat a day. Like me, you may struggle with this for a while. However, if you can turn the corner on meat consumption, you are on your way to a lifetime of weight control. If you doubt me, consider this: how many fat vegetarians do you know?

Duran-Thal emphasizes that the leanest cut of meat can become a fat dish if it is cooked by the wrong method. Meat should never be fried. Baking, broiling, grilling, microwaving, and stir-frying in a wok with very small amounts of cooking oil are the most healthful, lowest-fat ways to prepare meat, so retire the frying pan.

Most people underestimate the size of the portion they are eating and thus underestimate their daily calorie intake. Don't think an entree in a restaurant is a normal serving size. Most are double and sometimes even triple what is considered a normal serving for calorie counters. For instance, a cup of cooked pasta (without the sauce) is about 200 calories, but many restaurants serve triple that. Add the sauce and do the math and you can see that you could be eating over half of your daily calorie limit in just one dish.

Carol and I live about ten minutes from one of those mega-buffets where for $6.95 you can eat till you drop. Its customers, mostly obese, waddle in and fill their plates with lumberjack portions—several times. Eating more complex carbohydrates (vegetables, fruits, and whole grains) is the way to eat larger portions and not blow your calorie count.

INSTANT MATH

Figuring fat as a percentage of total calories is fairly simple, yet I sometimes find myself in the grocery store trying to do instant math and becoming frustrated. Kathy Duran-Thal has figured all the food options up to 19 grams of fat and 620 calories per serving in Figure 8.2. You won't be carrying this book to the store with you, so I suggest you make a copy of this table to put in your purse or wallet for easy reference.

A lot of busy working people eat microwavable dinners several times a week. Most of these dinners are about 300 to 400 calories, but many are loaded with fat. Start checking them with

FIGURE 8.2

FAT AS A PERCENTAGE OF TOTAL CALORIES

GRAMS OF FAT

CALORIES	1	2	3	4	5	6	7	8	9	10	11	12	13	14	15	16	17	18	19
150	.06	.12	.18	.24	.30	.36	.42	.48	.54	.60	.66	.72	.78	.84	.90	.96			
160	.05	.11	.16	.22	.28	.33	.39	.45	.50	.56	.61	.67	.73	.78	.84	.90	.95		
170	.05	.10	.15	.21	.26	.31	.37	.42	.47	.52	.58	.63	.68	.74	.79	.84	.90	.95	
180	.05	.10	.15	.20	.25	.30	.35	.40	.45	.50	.55	.60	.65	.70	.75	.80	.85	.90	.95
190	.04	.09	.14	.18	.23	.28	.33	.37	.42	.47	.52	.56	.61	.66	.71	.75	.80	.85	.90
200	.04	.09	.13	.18	.22	.27	.31	.36	.40	.45	.49	.54	.58	.63	.67	.72	.76	.81	.85
210	.04	.08	.12	.17	.21	.25	.30	.34	.38	.42	.47	.51	.55	.60	.64	.68	.72	.77	.81
220	.04	.08	.12	.16	.20	.24	.28	.32	.36	.40	.45	.49	.53	.57	.61	.65	.69	.73	.77
230	.03	.07	.11	.15	.19	.23	.27	.31	.35	.39	.43	.46	.50	.54	.58	.62	.66	.70	.74
240	.03	.07	.11	.15	.18	.22	.26	.30	.33	.37	.41	.45	.48	.52	.56	.60	.63	.67	.71
250	.03	.07	.10	.14	.18	.21	.25	.28	.32	.36	.39	.43	.46	.50	.54	.57	.61	.64	.68
260	.03	.06	.10	.13	.17	.20	.24	.27	.31	.34	.38	.41	.45	.48	.51	.55	.58	.62	.65
270	.03	.06	.10	.13	.16	.20	.23	.26	.30	.33	.36	.40	.43	.46	.50	.53	.56	.60	.63
280	.03	.06	.09	.12	.16	.19	.22	.25	.28	.32	.35	.38	.41	.45	.48	.51	.54	.57	.61
290	.03	.06	.09	.12	.15	.18	.21	.24	.27	.31	.34	.37	.40	.43	.46	.49	.52	.55	.58
300	.03	.06	.09	.12	.15	.18	.21	.24	.27	.30	.33	.36	.39	(42)	.45	.48	.51	.54	.57
310	.02	.05	.08	.11	.14	.17	.20	.23	.26	.29	.31	.34	.37	.40	.43	.46	.49	.52	.55
320	.02	.05	.08	.11	.14	.16	.19	.22	.25	.28	.30	.33	.36	.39	.42	.45	.47	.50	.53
330	.02	.05	.08	.10	.13	.16	.19	.21	.24	.27	.30	.32	.35	.38	.40	.43	.46	.49	.51
340	.02	.05	.07	.10	.13	.15	.18	.21	.23	.26	.29	.31	.34	.37	.39	.42	.45	.47	.50
350	.02	.05	.07	.10	.12	.15	.18	.20	.23	.25	.28	.30	.33	.36	.38	.41	.43	.46	.48
360	.02	.05	.07	.10	.12	.15	.17	.20	.22	.25	.27	.30	.32	.35	.37	.40	.42	.45	.47
370	.02	.04	.07	.09	.12	.14	.17	.19	.21	.24	.26	.29	.31	.34	.36	.38	.41	.43	.46
380	.02	.04	.07	.09	.11	.14	.16	.18	.21	.23	.26	.28	.30	.33	.35	.37	.40	.42	.45
390	.02	.04	.06	.09	.11	.13	.16	.18	.20	.23	.25	.27	.30	.32	.34	.36	.39	.41	.43
400	.02	.04	.06	.09	.11	.13	.15	.18	.20	.22	.24	.27	.29	.31	.33	.36	.38	.40	.42
410	.02	.04	.06	.08	.10	.13	.15	.17	.19	.21	.24	.26	.28	.30	.32	.35	.37	.39	.41
420	.02	.04	.06	.08	.10	.12	.15	.17	.19	.21	.23	.25	.27	.30	.32	.34	.36	.38	.40
430	.02	.04	.06	.08	.10	.12	.14	.16	.18	.20	.23	.25	.27	.29	.31	.33	.35	.37	.39
440	.02	.04	.06	.08	.10	.12	.14	.16	.18	.20	.22	.24	.26	.28	.30	.32	.34	.36	.38
450	.02	.04	.06	.08	.10	.12	.14	.16	.18	.20	.22	.24	.26	.28	.30	.32	.34	.36	.38
460	.01	.03	.05	.07	.09	.11	.13	.15	.17	.19	.21	.23	.25	.27	.29	.31	.33	.35	.37
470	.01	.03	.05	.07	.09	.11	.13	.15	.17	.19	.21	.22	.24	.26	.28	.30	.32	.34	.36
480	.01	.03	.05	.07	.09	.11	.13	.15	.16	.18	.20	.22	.24	.26	.28	.30	.31	.33	.35
490	.01	.03	.05	.07	.09	.11	.12	.14	.16	.18	.20	.22	.23	.25	.27	.29	.31	.33	.34
500	.01	.03	.05	.07	.09	.10	.12	.14	.16	.18	.19	.21	.23	.25	.27	.28	.30	.32	.34
510	.01	.03	.05	.07	.08	.10	.12	.14	.15	.17	.19	.21	.22	.24	.26	.28	.30	.31	.33
520	.01	.03	.05	.06	.08	.10	.12	.13	.15	.17	.19	.20	.22	.24	.25	.27	.29	.31	.32
530	.01	.03	.05	.06	.08	.10	.11	.13	.15	.16	.18	.20	.22	.23	.25	.27	.28	.30	.32
540	.01	.03	.05	.06	.08	.10	.11	.13	.15	.16	.18	.20	.21	.23	.25	.26	.28	.30	.31
550	.01	.03	.04	.06	.08	.09	.11	.13	.14	.16	.18	.19	.21	.22	.24	.26	.27	.29	.31
560	.01	.03	.04	.06	.08	.09	.11	.12	.14	.16	.17	.19	.20	.22	.24	.25	.27	.28	.30
570	.01	.03	.04	.06	.07	.09	.11	.12	.14	.15	.17	.18	.20	.22	.23	.25	.26	.28	.30
580	.01	.03	.04	.06	.07	.09	.10	.12	.13	.15	.17	.18	.20	.21	.23	.24	.26	.27	.29
590	.01	.03	.04	.06	.07	.09	.10	.12	.13	.15	.16	.18	.19	.21	.22	.24	.25	.27	.28
600	.01	.03	.04	.06	.07	.09	.10	.12	.13	.15	.16	.18	.19	.21	.22	.24	.25	.27	.28
610	.01	.02	.04	.05	.07	.08	.10	.11	.13	.14	.16	.17	.19	.20	.22	.23	.25	.26	.28
620	.01	.02	.04	.05	.07	.08	.10	.11	.13	.14	.15	.17	.18	.20	.21	.23	.24	.26	.27

© 1986 by Kathleen Sullivan Duran, dietitian

this table. For instance, if you bought a 300-calorie microwavable dinner with 14 grams of fat, it would have 42 percent fat calories (see the circle on the table). Try to buy a 300-calorie microwavable dinner with no more than 10 fat grams (30 percent fat) and preferably closer to 7 (21 percent fat).

WHEN IS LOW-FAT MILK NOT LOW-FAT?

For years people bought milk labeled "2 percent low-fat" because they wanted to cut down on their fat intake and believed that "2 percent low-fat" indicated that 98 percent of the fat was removed. Isn't that what you thought? You don't suppose the wholesome, squeaky-clean dairy industry would play labeling games with us, do you? I'll bet you a Holstein cow they would. What if the milk carton read "only 3.3 percent fat"? Wouldn't you also assume that 96.7 percent of the fat had been removed? Wrong. That's Elsie's full load of fat! The milk industry quotes fat as a percentage of weight instead of a percentage of calories. You will see in Figure 8.3 that 3.3 percent is all the fat there is in whole milk—by weight. In the fat column in Figure 8.3, you will see that 2 percent milk has 4.7 fat grams and whole milk 8.2. A nutrition label on a milk carton reveals that the 2 percent milk rounds the 4.7 up to 5 grams and the whole milk 8.2 down to 8. (The USDA permits rounding fractions to the nearest whole number.)

Four years ago the FDA made the milk processors quit that labeling deception and change "low-fat" to "reduced-fat" on 2 percent milk. It still has 5 grams of fat, however, and from a health and weight standpoint it is not a good choice for your diet. Skim milk, on the other hand, has the fewest calories, the least fat grams, and, as shown on the chart, the highest calcium

FIGURE 8.3

Type of Milk	Calories (per cup)	Fat (grams)	Calcium (milligrams)
Skim milk	86	0.4	302
Buttermilk, cultured	99	2.2	285
1% milk	102	2.6	300
2% milk	121	4.7	297
Whole milk, 3.3% fat	150	8.2	291
Chocolate milk, 2% fat	179	5.0	284
Chocolate milk, whole	208	8.5	280

Source: Agriculture Handbook No. 8–1, USDA Composition of Foods, Dairy and Egg Products.

content—a winning trifecta. If you are drinking 2 percent or whole milk, skim may seem thin and somewhat lacking in taste at first. If it does, switch to 1 percent or mix skim half and half with 2 percent. Over time you can train your taste buds to love skim milk.

Cutting fat from your diet means practically eliminating cheese. I confess that if there was one food that I could have in unlimited amounts, cheese would be it. Melted on various foods, added to a sandwich, or simply eaten with crackers, cheese hits my dietary hot button. Unfortunately, fat as a percentage of calories in a serving of cheese ranges from 60 to 85 percent. It is also mostly saturated fat, which is a negative for cholesterol and heart disease. Most of the fat-free cheeses taste like gum erasers unless melted on something; then they are passable—barely. The exception is Kraft's fat-free cream cheese. It's good!

The foregoing example of deception and hidden fat in a milk label was to illustrate that products you may have been consuming most of your life may not be what what you think they are. Buying any kind of processed food involves a risk of ending up with hidden fat that you don't need and didn't want. Ignore all the big, eye-catching numbers and phrases on the front of the package. Go right to the nutrition label and check the portion size and number of calories per serving. Look for the fat grams and compute the percentage of fat calories that the product has per serving. If it is over 30 percent, you should think long and hard about whether to buy it.

TRAINING THE TASTE BUDS

Eating smart is a process of reeducation. We all have taste preferences, and the daily decision-making process about what we will and won't eat is played out on our taste buds. We learned early in life that sweet is good, and that sweet coupled with fat (chocolate cake, cheesecake, etc.) is doubly good. Not only that, but sweet and fat were often elevated as a food choice by offering them as a reward. I can still remember my mother saying, "Eat your carrots or you won't get any butterscotch pie" (my favorite as a kid). Is there anyone who hasn't heard that kind of ultimatum?

Regardless of how old you are, most of your taste preferences for sweet, fat-laden foods were established at an early age, and the same taste-learning process continues for children today. Unfortunately, because of junk foods and high-fat school lunches (as well as lack of exercise), childhood obesity is a national problem. Pizza and highly sugared sodas are the favorites of most teenagers. These young taste buds are getting hooked early on the sweet-fat connection. That preference will be difficult for them to shake as they age, and for many their weight is already out of control.

Reeducating yourself to enjoy foods that are less fatty and less sweet is not something that you should do abruptly. Cutting out everything you like is what restrictive diets are all about. Ultimately they fail because the weight goal is reached by temporarily altering normal eating choices. Most people can psych themselves up and keep their taste buds under control for a while in order to lose a certain number of pounds. But part of that resolve comes from knowing that the diet is only temporary.

As we've seen, Oprah Winfrey did just that. She lived on a calorie-restricted liquid diet just long enough to fit into size-10 jeans. Then, slowly but surely, her taste buds drew her back to her favorite foods, such as mashed potatoes made with butter and horseradish, and key lime pie, according to *People* magazine. What happened to Oprah has happened to me at least a half dozen times. I sympathize with her and know what a helpless feeling it is to crave a certain food—almost like an alcoholic craves a drink or a heavy smoker needs a cigarette.

The challenge we all face is to reduce calories and fat intake while satisfying our taste buds. Most flavor preferences are learned (usually culturally), but a couple are inborn. For instance, babies prefer sweet flavors from birth, and bitterness is universally disliked from birth. Bitter foods, such as black coffee or quinine water, can become an acquired taste. If you make a concerted effort to reeducate your taste buds to like certain foods and liquids that are good for you, you will eat and drink them more often. It should be a gradual process, however.

In the Western industrialized countries, and in particular the United States, meat and dairy products are introduced into our diets early, and our taste buds get hooked on them. In other countries, taste preferences develop for totally different foods. China, for instance, does not have a large dairy industry, so milk and butter are rare. In fact, the Chinese call butter "cow oil" and consider its taste repugnant. The eating habits we learn as young children create an "indelible blueprint for adult behavior patterns," according to Kathy Duran-Thal.

People who want to control their weight and eat nutritiously must also retrain their minds. Meat and high-fat dairy products should be deemphasized in favor of whole grains, vegetables, fruits, and low-fat dairy products. We must unlearn some of our early beliefs about why we need to eat a lot of meat protein and ingest a lot of dairy products for calcium. There are other, more healthful ways to get adequate protein and calcium. Today's typical diet in Western industrialized countries is much higher in animal fat and protein than we need or should have, and this raises the risks of cancer, heart disease, obesity, diabetes, and osteoporosis. There has been an overemphasis on protein (i.e., meat); studies show that the average American eats about twice as much as needed.

THE PREHISTORIC DIET

In *The Paleolithic Prescription* (now out of print), Dr. S. Boyd Eaton, Marjorie Shostak, and Dr. Melvin Konner analyze the dietary intake and lifestyles of our ancestors of forty thousand years ago, when the human species were hunter-gatherers. This was before the advent of agriculture and domesticated animals. A persuasive case is made that we should blend the best dietary and exercise features from the past with the best from the present.

The authors point out that between 1910 and 1976 consumption of fats in the United States increased by about 25 percent, so that today fat makes up about 42 percent on average of the calories we consume each day. They state, "This level of fat consumption is unprecedented in human evolutionary experience and results in diseases that kill us, but that are uncommon in countries where fat represents a much smaller portion of the diet." The diet in rural Japan is cited. Only 10 to 12 percent of the daily calories come from fat, and the prevalence of coronary heart disease among rural Japanese is just a fraction of ours. Recent studies show, however, that when Japanese move to Western industrialized countries and increase their fat intake, they also evidence an increase in heart disease.

It is difficult for us to realize that the ten thousand years since agriculture and domesticated animals came on the scene is only an instant in terms of our total evolutionary development. It took millions of years to develop our upright bipedal locomotion system. Our physical activity requirements and dietary needs were being developed at the same time. Now, in just a few years by evolutionary standards, we have nearly eliminated significant physical activity and drastically altered the composition and quantity of food that we eat. This has played havoc with the way we accumulate and store fat. The authors of *The Paleolithic Prescription* point out that the fat-storage pattern of free-living mammals other than humans is fairly uniform. For instance, have you ever noticed in some of the TV documentaries that a herd of zebras or wildebeests on the plains of Africa all look as if they weigh about the same? The deer and coyotes that frequently pass through my rural acreage are also uniform in size. As the authors state, "The range of body composition in wild animal species is relatively narrow."

As we human animals got smarter, we learned how to produce a year-round supply of food. The hunter-gatherer life of our prehistoric ancestors became obsolete, and as a result, our body composition changed from what was once a moderately uniform range to an extreme one. Now body fat can account for between 2 and 60 percent of our total weight, according to Eaton, Shostak, and Konner. Unlike wild animals, humans similar in age, height, and sex differ widely in the amount of fat they carry.

The unlimited amount of high-density fat calories available in most Western countries, with so little physical effort needed to obtain them, makes excess fat an inevitable consequence. A few centuries ago, only the wealthy were fat, but now that condition has reversed. Obesity is a hallmark of the lower socioeconomic level, while many of the educated and well-to-do have the knowledge and desire to maintain a healthier weight range. As *The Paleolithic Prescription* points out, "This transfer of obesity to the poor is occurring at the same time as obesity's harmful health effects are becoming well documented."

Stone Age people were lean, strong, aerobically fit, and almost totally free from the chronic diseases that cause 75 percent of all deaths in the United States today. It should be noted, however, that Stone Age people's life expectancy was considerably less than ours because they died of diseases that have since been eradicated by modern medicine. The authors state: "Our genetic make-up—designed over millions of years and largely unchanged in the last ten thousand—has become sharply discordant with life today; drastic changes in human nutrition and exercise patterns have promoted cancer, heart disease, diabetes, hypertension, obesity, and even tooth decay." Clearly, being overfed and underexercised contributes to poor health and lessened longevity.

If you are seriously overweight, health is the primary and

maybe the *only* reason you should lose weight, because fat culls the human herd quietly and quickly. Obituaries don't list fatness as the cause of death, but we now know that it produces a friendly environment for adult diabetes, some cancers, heart disease, and hypertension. Such diseases are listed on the official death record, but excess fat is the silent, lethal accomplice. What is your mirror telling you to do?

CURBING YOUR APPETITE

You know you should cut back on the amount you eat to shed those extra pounds, but sometimes it seems impossible. Here are a few tips that may help you curb your appetite and avoid overeating from the September 2005 *Mayo Clinic Health Letter.* They are:

- *Don't skip breakfast.* If you make breakfast a high-fiber cereal, whole-grain bread, or fresh fruit, you will be less likely to overeat at lunch.
- *Eat slowly.* Savor each flavor and texture and remember it takes about 20 minutes for your brain to receive the signal that you are full.
- *Think small.* If you always eat everything that is on your plate, start with half the amount of food you usually eat. And, to make less food seem like more, have your main course on a salad plate or dessert plate.
- *Eat only when you are hungry.* Stop and ask yourself whether you are stressed or bored or truly hungry. Then act accordingly.
- *Ride out the urge.* Cravings generally pass within seconds or minutes. Engage in an activity unrelated to food until

the desire to eat passes. Exercise is an especially good—and healthy—distraction.

• *Allow an occasional splurge.* If you are really committed to eating less, an occasional lapse is fine. In the long run, it will have little impact on your lifetime plan for controlling your appetite.

I not only practice all of those tips, I would like to expand on a few. All of the healthful advice I have ever read says that breakfast is the most important meal of the day, and I never skip breakfast. There is an old saying that you should "eat breakfast like a king, lunch like a prince, and dinner like a pauper." Most people practice that backward. Get up a few minutes earlier in the morning and allow time for a hearty, nutritious breakfast to start your day. If you are going to lighten up on calories, do it at the evening meal.

I had to learn to eat slowly, but it is worth learning. When I was growing up my father would inhale his dinner in about nine minutes; consequently, our meals were quite brief. With that background, I tended to wolf down everything without truly savoring the flavors, textures, and aromas of the food. Eating slowly allows you to reach satiety, which takes about 20 minutes.

If you have ever eaten in a very busy restaurant and it took over 30 minutes to get your entree after you have had your salad, a roll, and possibly a glass of wine, chances are you weren't very hungry when the main course arrived. The entree doesn't seem nearly as appealing as when you first sat down because you have reached satiety. Don't stuff yourself; take part of the entree home in a doggy bag. Also, *never* eat standing up, particularly at the kitchen counter. Even if you are only having a snack, put a portion on a plate and sit down and enjoy it. Otherwise, you will just be hurriedly taking on calories without any real enjoyment.

The only reason to eat is if you are genuinely hungry. Eating because you are stressed, angry, happy, or experiencing any feeling other than hunger leads to bingeing and finding excuses to use food as a mental crutch. And it leads to obesity. I was guilty of that so many times I am ashamed to admit it. Conquering emotional eating is one of the first battles everyone must win to be successful in a long-term weight management program.

Finally, mastering random cravings that can hit you at anytime of the day (and sometimes night) requires resolve and usually physical action. My weakness is something crunchy and salty, such as cashews or potato chips. Others may crave chocolate or ice cream, but whatever it is, remember, it is mostly *mental* and not actual hunger. Generally speaking, we tend to crave dessert or snack-type foods as opposed to main course foods. I don't know anybody who ever had a craving for broccoli or turnips.

You may never totally lose the occasional craving (I never did), but you can control it. I get out of the house for a short walk, read an interesting article, or run an errand. The important thing is to do something physically and/or mentally until the urge passes.

CASEY'S RANDOM TIPS ON FIGHTING FAT

Over the last 20 years or so I have learned a number of things about eating smart that help make the fat fight a breeze. Here are a few ideas that work for me and may help you.

Grazing

I picked this idea up in *Jane Brody's Good Food Book*. (She didn't call it grazing, but the principle is the same.) Eat five or six small, low-fat meals throughout the day instead of two or three big ones. Our prehistoric ancestors were grazers; they were constantly moving about trying to find food. Only in modern times do we sit down at prescribed times to eat. Drink a full glass of water before each snack, and you will rarely be hungry. (This also helps you get your necessary water intake.) Sometimes I eat three bowls of cereal in the course of a day, with fresh fruit, fat-free milk, and Splenda. It drives Carol nuts, but I think cereal and fruit make a great low-fat dessert!

Yogurt-Cereal Lunch

My favorite lunch is a no-fat fruit yogurt (100 calories or less) over any fresh fruit in season (preferably blueberries) with a tablespoon of Grape-Nuts sprinkled over it. The Grape-Nuts taste great and add a crunchy texture. Stir this up, and you will have a delicious, healthful lunch. You are getting calcium, whole grains, antioxidants, no fat, and about 200 calories, and you will feel full. Bananas are always available; add one and you are also getting potassium.

Forget the Butter

I have not had butter or margarine on bread or toast in over twenty years. At breakfast I usually top a piece of Carol's toasted homemade seven-grain bread with strawberry preserves. Learn to leave the butter or margarine off and reduce your saturated fat intake. Preserves or jelly has only about 18 calories per teaspoon and zero saturated fat. Your taste buds won't miss the butter because they will love the taste of jelly. Preserves, honey, jelly, and apple butter are great substitutes for butter or margarine. A few calories of sugar are a better trade-off than a lot of artery-clogging saturated fat.

Crunchy and Salty

I get the craving for something crunchy and salty once in a while. Frito-Lay makes potato chips and tortilla chips with a fake fat called Olestra. The potato chips have zero fat and half the calories of regular chips. The tortilla chips have one third fewer calories than regular tortilla chips and only one gram of fat, which is from the corn. I think both chips taste great. In fact, I can't tell the difference (and I am a tough sell) from those loaded with saturated fat and a lot of calories. Look for them in a light blue package with the word "Light" in large letters on the front. It is a guilt-free way to satisfy a craving for something crunchy and salty—but don't go overboard. Pretzels are also a way to satisfy that kind of craving, rather than salty peanuts, which are high in fat and calories. There are several makes of pretzels that are fat-free and taste as good as the others. Read the labels to be safe.

New Potatoes

We all have the need for crunchy food from time to time. That's why liquid diets soon become a problem. New potatoes are small red- or tan-skinned potatoes. Wash three or four that are not much bigger than an oversized English walnut and eat them raw as you would an apple, skin and all. They are crunchy, delicious, and nutritious. If you don't have a sodium problem, sprinkle a little salt on them. Four small potatoes have about 100 calories and no fat calories. Try it, you might like it.

Portion Control

I win lots of bets with Carol on what a portion is. We bring out our kitchen scale, which weighs in grams and ounces, and weigh a portion. She generally has dished out enough to feed a lumberjack, so we cut it down in size. As I've noted, most people underestimate portion sizes and end up eating much more than they realize. If you are in a serious weight loss or weight maintenance program, next to exercise there is nothing more important than portion control. You can't be a winner without it. A small, accurate kitchen scale is a good investment and will help you train your eye to judge portion sizes.

The Two-Bite Dessert

At the end of a good meal sometimes the desire for a sweet (usually fat-heavy) dessert becomes irresistible. If you turn it down, chances are you will still be thinking about it at 3 a.m. Here's my solution. At a restaurant, Carol and I mutually agree on a dessert, and order one with two forks. We limit ourselves to two normal bites. I eat mine very slowly and keep it on my tongue as long as possible, letting it dissolve like a piece of hard candy. This gives my taste buds the sugar and fat fix they were screaming for, yet I have only eaten a small amount of fat calories. I have satisfied my craving. By limiting yourself to two normal bites, you also reinforce your discipline. Just as important, you will feel a lot better than if you ate the whole portion and then wished you hadn't. How many times have we all done that?

Blender Smoothies

I have fun tossing various fruits into a blender to see what they taste like. One of my favorites is a cup of ice cubes, a cup of orange juice, any nonfat fruit yogurt, a banana, a few frozen strawberries, frozen blueberries, and a packet of Splenda. Run the blender until everything is thoroughly blended, pour it in a large glass, and grate nutmeg on top. If it is too thick to pour easily, add a little water or more orange juice. This is tastier than a milkshake, loaded with antioxidants, and very filling without any fat calories. In the frozen food section of your supermarket you can usually find big bags of strawberries and fruit combinations that are cheaper than fresh fruit.

For a 79-year-old retired businessman to be giving you tips about nutrition and weight control is proof positive that the learning process in life never quits; that's what keeps us young beyond our years. There was a time I wouldn't even try a lot of fruits and vegetables. I was a meat-and-potatoes guy, and everything I ate had to be fatty, sweet, or both. Now nothing goes in my mouth unless I know that it is good for me. This old guy wants to remain healthy and live to be a lot older. At my age I don't have a lot of wiggle room, so I have changed my eating pattern from gluttonous gratification to smart eating. Give it a chance. Eating smart works for me, and it will work for you too. But don't forget your daily walk.

GET INFORMED AND STAY INFORMED

Knowledge about nutrition and healthful eating is a moving target. New studies and new information about the role certain foods play in our diets are coming out all of the time. The more you read and understand about how your body functions and the fuel it needs, the easier it will be for you to maintain proper weight and a healthy lifestyle. With the advent of the Internet and the availability of instant, accurate information, anyone can be up to date with the click of a mouse. For those who don't have a computer there are a number of publications that provide reliable exercise, health, diet, and nutrition information. Here are the publications I take and the websites that I have found to be reliable:

University of California at Berkeley Wellness Letter
Subscription Department
P.O. Box 420148
Palm Coast, FL 32142
800-829-9170
www.WellnessLetter.com

I have taken this letter for over 20 years and look forward to it every month. It is easy to read and covers nutrition, exercise, and all subjects related to wellness.

Tufts University Health & Nutrition Letter
Subscription Department
P.O. Box 420235
Palm Coast, FL 32142
800-274-7581
www.healthletter.tufts.edu

This fine letter focuses on diet, nutrition, and health issues. Their masthead motto is: "Your Guide to Living Healthier Longer."

Mayo Clinic Health Letter
Subscription Services
P.O. Box 9302
Big Sandy, TX 75755
www.MayoClinic.com

Published by the internationally famous Mayo Clinic, this letter will keep you informed about the many aspects of proper nutrition and health.

The Johns Hopkins Medical Letter—Health After 50
P.O. Box 420179
Palm Coast, FL 32142
www.hopkinsafter50.com

For baby boomers, this excellent health letter published by the prestigious Johns Hopkins Medical Center is a must.

Don't be intimidated by health and nutrition letters from universities or places such as the Mayo Clinic or Johns Hopkins. They are written in layman's language and easily read. Their websites are excellent and provide a wide range of information.

Other websites that I have found to be reliable and informative on health and health-related regulatory issues are:

Centers for Disease Control and Prevention
    www.cdc.gov
U.S. Food and Drug Administration
    www.fda.gov

National Institutes of Health
www.nih.gov
American Heart Association
www.americanheart.org
National Cancer Institute
www.cancer.gov
American Dietetic Association
www.eatright.org
Health Fraud and Quackery
www.quackwatch.com
Fit Day (calculate daily intake)
www.fitday.com
Meals.com
www.meals.com
Zoom Cafe (kids will love this)
www.pbskids.org/zoom/cafe
American Council on Science and Health
www.acsh.org
President's Council on Physical Fitness and Sports
www.fitness.gov
U.S. Soyfoods Directory
www.soyfoods.com
New England Journal of Medicine
www.nejm.org
American Medical Association
www.ama-assn.org
American Diabetes Association
www.diabetes.org
National Heart, Lung, and Blood Institute
www.nhlbi.nih.gov
American Weight Control Registry
www.lifespan.org

WebMD
www.webmd.com

To give you the inspiration to take charge of your life with exercise and diet, I can't think of a better living example to close this chapter with than Rick Salewske, the weight loss champ (lost 300 pounds) in the *People* magazine story I mentioned earlier. When I saw that he got his start at the Cooper Aerobics Center run by Dr. Kenneth Cooper, I contacted one of my friends there, who put me in touch with him. Salewske willingly told his phenomenal weight loss story to me so I could share it with you.

Salewske went from 538 pounds to 238 in two years. He hit his weight goal in October 2002 and is holding firm at that weight as this is being written in January of 2006. The first four months Salewske worked with a personal trainer and nutritionist at the Cooper Aerobics Center. By then he had lost 100 pounds but still had 200 to go. He continues to have a 30-minute workout once a week with the personal trainer. Salewske was barely able to walk one-eighth of a mile on his first day, but a year later he could run 7 miles consistently, had lost 230 pounds, and completed a half-marathon—remarkable. He lost the final 70 pounds in the second year.

Besides an aggressive exercise regimen during weight loss, Salewske's diet went from fast food to lots of fruit, vegetables, fish, chicken, low-fat milk, and bran cereal, totaling 1,500 calories a day. Now he eats about 2,000 calories a day, runs 45 to 60 minutes six days a week, and weighs himself every day. Salewske also does some weight training two to three times a week to build muscle, which helps him burn more calories.

Salewske runs because he had never heard of aerobic walking. He is forty-three, and at 6 feet 1 inch tall and big-boned, he realizes that someday injury may stop his running. I took the opportunity to get a future walking disciple and sent him a copy of the first edition of *Walking*.

As the weight came off, Salewske said his blood pressure came down, his cholesterol came down, and his confidence went up. Since his weight loss, he has gotten married, and two weeks before we talked he became the proud father of a baby boy.

Salewske's weight loss and weight maintenance schedule are similar to mine and those of every person I know who successfully controls his or her weight. It always hinges on the premise of calories in and calories out. A caloric deficit must be established during weight loss and caloric equilibrium during weight maintenance.

One other vital aspect is necessary for success—mental commitment. Several times throughout our conversation Salewske said, "It is all mental." He is right. He had made up his mind that he was going to lose the weight and that he would not fail. Salewske kept saying, "I knew I could do it." An unyielding mental commitment is the glue that holds a weight control program together. If you have a weight problem, be a winner and take charge of your weight and your health as Rick Salewske did. Now is the time to start walking and eating smart.

NINE

Shoes, Socks, Weather, Helpful Tips, and Frequently Asked Questions

SHOES

Not only did exercise-walking have to launch itself, but there was even a time when the necessity of an exercise-walking shoe was in doubt. "Do Exercise Walkers Need Special Walking Shoes?" was a feature article in the June 1987 issue of *The Physician and Sportsmedicine* magazine. Out of nowhere, exercise-walking had emerged and, as the article reported, it was not until 1986 that the National Sporting Goods Association (NSGA) gathered the first statistics on it. In its initial walking-activities survey, the association projected that there were 49.7

million exercise-walkers in the United States compared with an estimated 33.0 million joggers. The significance of this comparison is that jogging had been a popular, widely publicized aerobic exercise for over eight years, yet exercise-walking, still in its infancy, had already taken the lead by a wide margin.

Fast-forward to January 2006. On the NSGA's website, the "Ten Year History of Selected Sports Participation" showed that exercise-walking in 1994 comprised 70.8 percent of exercises and 84.7 percent in 2004. Running/jogging in 1994 was 20.6 percent and 24.7 percent in 2004. With such impressive numbers dating back to 1986, one would assume the shoe manufacturers would get interested in exercise-walking in a big way. They did, and by April 1991 *The Walking Magazine,* in its "Buyer's Guide" issue, featured fifty-seven models of exercise-walking shoes. Unfortunately, that was the high point of the evolution of the walking shoe, and it has been in decline since then.

The Walking Magazine is no longer in existence, and there are only a handful of companies that make walking shoes. In addition, many of the early walking "experts" advised that jogging shoes were good enough for walkers. There is some truth to that. A beginning walker who is possibly overweight and walking at the stroll pace will not be at an intensity level where a shoe will have much influence on the biomechanics of his or her gait.

Going back three million years to Lucy, bipedality has functioned quite well by walking and running without shoes. Even today in less-developed countries approximately two billion people spend their whole lives walking and running barefoot, or in nothing more than thong sandals. Empirical evidence indicates that they have fewer foot problems than those of us who wear shoes. An issue of the *University of California at Berkeley*

Wellness Letter observed, "Ill-fitting shoes, it is thought, cause 80 percent of all foot problems. Besides causing corns, bunions, nail deformities, and other problems, painful shoes can alter your gait and your outlook for the worse." Nevertheless, in Western industrialized countries we wear shoes, and there is a bewildering array of styles, colors, and models of athletic or exercise shoes to choose from. How do you choose the right one amidst all the marketing claims? A quick review of the differences between the biomechanics of the walking and running gaits will show you why a running shoe and some other models are counterproductive for an exercise-walker.

Features of a Good Walking Shoe

As you learned in Chapter 2, a runner is airborne on each step and hits the running surface with a force about three and a half times his or her body weight. The body's entire mass is loaded abruptly onto a single foot. Humans were not biomechanically engineered with an effective shock-absorbing system, so the running-shoe companies have tried to devise one by strapping a collision mat to the bottom of the foot. They have come up with all kinds of ingenious devices—airbags, gels, and tubings—designed to mask the shock of running and supposedly reduce injuries.

For instance, back in the mid-1980s, one of the early ads for the then new Nike Air Cushion Shoe showed an automobile crash test with an airbag deployed. The ad copy stated: "On average, you'll crash 17,600 times during a 10-mile trip. And with every single impact, shock waves will be sent tearing through your body at speeds up to 120 miles per hour. We're talking about running. And the most important reason you need Nike—

air cushioning." Does anybody, by the wildest stretch of the imagination, believe that a little airbag on the bottom of your foot could effectively absorb or dissipate that much shock to your musculoskeletal system?

Some shoe companies designed their running shoes for "damage control." That was the main theme of Etonic's ad campaign for its new running shoe in the April 1991 "Spring Shoe Buyer's Guide" of *Runner's World*. The first line of the ad read, "The damage report is in; 61.6% of all runners were injured last year." It is obvious that the airbags, gels, and other gimmicks cannot compensate for the basic fact that the human animal is not designed for frequent, prolonged running. The big, thick heel and squishy sole that act as a collision mat in Figure 9.1, which shows a generic running shoe, are counterproductive for the walking gait. In spite of marketing claims, they also don't seem to be effective in preventing running injuries. The walking gait lets the walker load his or her body weight onto the foot in a lower-impact, more gentle way. A walker does not need a defensive shoe, designed to absorb impact, but an offensive shoe that will permit the foot to function naturally in its most biomechanically efficient manner. In effect, an exercise-walking shoe's design should be exactly the opposite of a running shoe.

People buy dress shoes primarily because of the quality of leather, color, texture, and decorative design. In an exercise-walking shoe, however, it's what's under the foot that's more important. The way the walking platform of a shoe is designed from the heel, where the walking motion begins, to the toe, where the foot must bend for toe-off, determines how your foot will function. Anything that inhibits the natural motion of the foot, which functioned without shoes or sandals for thousands of years, will affect the foot's biomechanical efficiency. Your foot

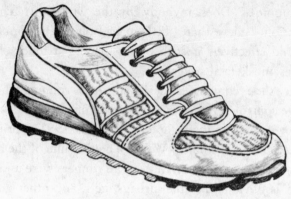

FIGURE 9.1

and the muscles in your legs will be fighting the restrictions of the shoe.

Heel elevation is a prime consideration in the walking motion. Dr. Verne Inman, who authored *Human Walking*, observed that women in high heels take shorter steps than do women in low heels. On the highly popular TV show *Sex and the City*, Sarah Jessica Parker made four-inch spiked heels and pointy toed shoes popular and sensual. However, when I did walking clinics I always asked the women what they did with their high-heeled shoes when they get home from work or a party. In unison they sang out, "Take 'em off!" The obvious reason, of course, is to get the heel back down where it belongs, in its most natural, comfortable position.

The primary role of the walking platform is to protect the bottom of the foot. This role has not changed since the first sandal was made several thousand years ago. In addition, the walking platform must provide moderate cushioning for comfort on our hard walking surfaces. Remember, there were no concrete, asphalt, or macadam roads until recent times. The evolution of the walking gait occurred on terra firma.

A good walking-shoe platform should provide adequate protection and the proper amount of cushioning without elevating the heel too far from its natural position, which distorts the walking motion. It is nearly impossible to get the right combination of cushioning and protection in a walking platform that is less than ½ inch thick at the heel. It is also apparent that, when the heel is elevated much beyond ¾ of an inch, it starts to alter the biomechanical efficiency of the foot. I prefer a heel closer to ½ inch, because I like to walk fast, and it is easier to do so in a lower heel.

High, overbuilt heels are a major reason jogging shoes are not good exercise-walking shoes. Another reason is that jogging shoes are too soft at the heel for a walker. When a walker loads his or her weight onto a jogging shoe's high, squishy heel, it continues to compress as the walker's weight comes down on the foot. This is a microversion of walking on sand. When you walk on the beach your heel continues to sink as you load your weight on it, and your leg muscles get tired quickly. Trying to walk fast in jogging shoes causes a similar fatigue. Admittedly, you can walk slowly in any kind of shoes—or with no shoes at all. A good exercise-walking shoe, however, should permit you to walk efficiently at the low-, moderate-, and high-intensity levels.

One of the early makers of exercise-walking shoes designed a walking platform that was about 1 inch high at the heel and rigid from the heel to the toe. The company called it a "rocker" design, and it was supposed to aid the walking motion. They sent me a pair. They were comfortable shoes at a slow stroll, but as I attempted the brisk pace the higher heel and rigid forefoot of the walking platform fought the natural movement of my foot and caused fatigue in my legs. It was like putting a governor on my foot, and I could not walk faster than a 15-minute mile without considerable leg stress.

A good exercise-walking shoe platform should not be stiff at the forefoot (the ball of the foot), as many jogging and cross-training shoes are. Rigid soles at the forefoot on exercise-walking shoes interfere with toe-off, which is an essential part of the foot's contribution to your forward progress and speed.

Dr. Inman's research in *Human Walking* addresses the way the foot reacts biomechanically from heel plant to toe-off. He states: "As the foot is loaded, it can be seen to pronate. As the heel is raised, there is a rapid but slight inversion of the heel as the foot supinates." The terms *pronate* and *supinate* are better understood visually than by a lengthy definition. Figure 9.2A shows a right pronating foot, and Figure 9.2B shows a right supinating foot.

You can see how your foot reacts when you load your weight onto it. Take your shoe and sock off one foot. With your foot slightly in front of you and your toes up, as if you were taking a short step, place your heel on the floor, slowly lower your fore-foot onto the floor, and bring your body over it. As your fore-foot comes down so that all your weight is evenly distributed on the whole foot, you will notice that your medial ankle area will bulge slightly and tend to roll to the inside (pronate). On most overweight or obese people, these tendencies are quite pronounced.

As you load your weight onto your forefoot and toes, notice how your forefoot widens and the middle toes tend to spread. When your heel rises as you start to toe off, observe how your foot shifts to the outside edge (supinates) as you transfer all your weight to the front of it. When the forefoot is in the last stages

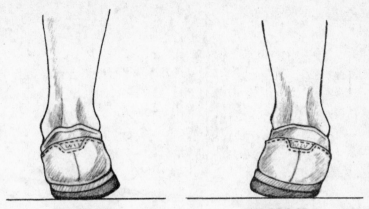

FIGURE 9.2A   FIGURE 9.2B

of flexing before toe-off, you will notice that it bends at an oblique angle just behind the toes. Dr. Inman calls this oblique angle between the toes and metatarsal bones the "metatarsophalangeal break."

The metatarsals are the big bones in the forefoot to which the phalanges (toes) are connected. Figure 9.3 shows the metatarsophalangeal angle in relation to the long axis of the foot. Dr. Inman points out: "To distribute the weight between all metatarsal heads, the foot must deviate laterally (supinate) at push-off."

Supple forefoot flex in an exercise-walking shoe is absolutely essential to accommodate the foot's natural bend at toe-off, as shown in Figure 9.3. Some rocker-type shoes, most cross-trainers, and jogging shoes are too rigid at this critical biomechanical juncture. They restrict the foot's ability to contribute to forward propulsion at toe-off and cause the foot to labor against the stiff walking platform as it tries to bend in its natural manner. An exercise-walker wearing such shoes and trying to accel-

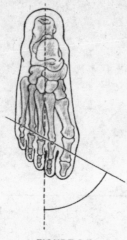

FIGURE 9.3

erate beyond the brisk pace will experience unnecessary shin fatigue and stress in the leg muscles.

A good exercise-walking shoe should have a comfortably wide toe box to accommodate the widening of the forefoot when the body weight is loaded onto it. The toe box should also be high enough to give the toes adequate clearance. Figure 9.4 shows a hypothetical generic walking shoe.

The platform of an exercise-walking shoe should be essentially neutral. It should not try to manage the foot's biomechanics but should let it move from heel plant to toe-off in its most natural manner. It should be just thick enough to protect the bottom of the foot, and provide a moderate amount of cushioning.

A variety of materials and constructions are used in the platforms of exercise-walking shoes. The most common combination is a molded platform consisting of a rubber outsole that

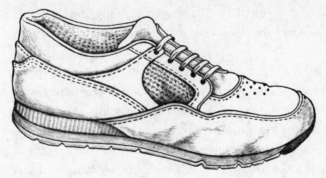

FIGURE 9.4

makes contact with the walking surface. The midsole is a cushioning material sandwiched between the outsole and the insole,
which is what the foot rests on inside the shoe. The uppers
should be made of breathable leather or a combination of nylon
mesh and leather. Good walking shoes have removable insole inserts that have a buildup arch control. These inserts can be removed to dry if wet from sweat.

How to Buy Walking Shoes

When you go shopping for exercise-walking shoes, do not assume the shoe clerk knows anything about walking as an exercise or how an exercise-walking shoe should differ from a
jogging shoe. My experience has been that most of the young
salespeople in athletic-shoe stores are more familiar with jogging/
running and are not knowledgeable about exercise-walking.
They are likely to recommend a so-called walking shoe made
by a major athletic-shoe company simply because they have
sold the company's running shoes and are familiar with the

brand name. You are probably getting a jogging shoe clone. You must be your own walking-shoe expert and know what to look for.

Here is the sequence to follow when buying the most important piece of equipment an exercise-walker needs: properly fitting walking shoes. Your buying decision should always be made on the basis of *fit and comfort* over any technical features. If the shoes don't fit right and feel good on your feet the moment you put them on, you won't be a happy walker. There is no break-in period for walking shoes.

The buying guidelines are:

- It is best to buy shoes at midday or later, or after you have had your daily walk. Feet may swell up to a half size over the course of the day.
- Always fit shoes wearing the kind of socks you walk in.
- Get both feet measured with the measuring device that shoe stores use when you buy shoes. Foot size can change, particularly if you have gained or lost a lot of weight. Additionally, almost all athletic shoes are made in Asia, and their sizes don't seem to match ours. I measure size 12 but have to buy size 13 exercise-walking shoes. Whatever your foot measures, be prepared to buy a size larger.
- Always stand and load your weight onto the foot being measured. Your forefoot widens when it is bearing weight.
- Put both shoes on and lace them up evenly. Some clerks leave the lower laces loose and merely snug them at the top eyelets. You need to know how the upper of the shoe forms to your entire foot and how it holds the walking platform in place. Take an extra few seconds and lace the shoes up evenly and snugly.

- *This is critical: walk in the shoes on a hard surface.* Department stores usually have a hard-surface aisle, and shopping malls are hard-surfaced outside the shoe store. Most people stand around on carpet trying to make a buying decision. They end up looking in the little mirror down on the floor to see if the shoes look attractive on their feet and buy them more for cosmetic reasons than for biomechanical functionality.
- On a hard surface, walk ten or fifteen steps at your fastest pace; do so back and forth several times. Check how your weight is loaded onto the foot at heel plant and how your foot rolls forward to toe-off. Is the shoe flexible in the forefoot? Is there rubbing or tightness anywhere? Is the toe box wide enough? Is there looseness at the heel? Walking at your fastest pace lets your foot interact with the shoe and the walking surface to bring out any deficiencies. Most shoes feel pretty good when you are standing on a carpet or just taking a few slow steps. The acid test for a walking shoe is to put your foot in action on a hard surface, just as you do on your daily walk. I recommend that you walk-check regular dress shoes the same way. You'll be surprised how quickly you can eliminate ill-fitting shoes before buying them.
- Many people have one foot a bit longer than the other. Always accommodate the longer foot when sizing. Allow at least ¼ inch of clearance between your toe and the end of the toe box. If you walk-check the shoe thoroughly, you will find out at toe-off whether you have adequate clearance.
- Check the forefoot area for flex. Can you take the shoe in your hand and easily bend it to the angle at which your

foot naturally bends at toe-off? If not, the shoe will fight your foot as you try to walk at the brisk pace or faster.

An exception to this rule is a hiking shoe. Of necessity it will have a stiffer, thicker sole for protection of the foot in off-pavement walking. Hiking is much slower than brisk-paced walking, and toe-off action is minimal. The theoretical exercise-walking shoe described earlier was meant for low-, moderate-, and high-intensity exercise walking on smooth, paved surfaces. A shoe that functions well on this kind of surface will lack the protection and rigidity for walking on uneven, off-pavement surfaces. If you hike, you should have hiking shoes that can accommodate those conditions.

I have described an ideal exercise-walking shoe, but unfortunately, I do not know of a shoe company that makes such a shoe. All of the "walking shoes" I have found are jogging shoe clones and to me are unacceptable for a serious walker. In the mid-eighties Nike made a gray walking shoe for about a year that was like the one I described and it was superb! Perhaps their timing was too early and they quit making it. If they brought it back now I would buy it in a heartbeat.

In the meantime, I suggest that you go to the casual-shoe section in a major sporting goods or athletic-shoe store and look for a low-heeled, light, flexible casual shoe. This type of shoe has more of the right walking shoe characteristics than their "walking shoes." If you are extremely overweight, however, a major brand "walking shoe" will work for you until you lose some weight. You will be walking at an entry-level stroll and the walking platform will not impede your foot action.

If you don't have any luck at a local athletic-shoe store, here is another option. I currently buy my walking shoes from Eastbay. They are a huge shoe and athletic equipment source at www.eastbay.com or 800-826-2205. Their catalog and website have the largest casual shoe section I have ever found. It is not ideal to buy from a picture, but if you know your size (example: American size 10 would be an Asian 11) and you see a shoe with a low heel by a big brand name such as Adidas, Puma, Nike, or Reebok, it will probably handle any walking pace you need. If it doesn't, Eastbay has a very good return policy.

BEWARE OF WALKING-SHOE "BARGAINS"

Buying the lowest-priced shoe may cause you to pay a higher price later in foot and other problems. At 2006 prices, a good pair of exercise-walking shoes (or casual shoes) will cost between $60 and $90. Some national discount stores advertise athletic-looking shoes for less than $30, but they have cheap composition material in the midsoles that mashes down and often aggravates pronation.

A middle-aged woman at one of my walking clinics told me she was starting to have knee and back discomfort after her daily walks. I checked her shoes. They weren't worn out; in fact, they looked as if they had just come out of the box. They had a generic look, and I didn't recognize them by make. I asked her where she'd gotten them, how long she'd had them, and how much she'd paid for them. She had bought them from one of the leading discount stores, had worn them for eight weeks, and proudly proclaimed that they cost only $23. Her discomfort had started about three weeks after buying those shoes.

I got behind her and asked her to walk away from me at her fastest pace. In only a few steps, I could see that she was pronating badly as she loaded her weight onto her foot at heel plant. I then had her take both shoes off and walk away from me again. She hardly pronated at all. The midsoles of her shoes had mashed down on the medial side, creating a situation like a slanted sidewalk, so that every time she took a step her foot came down in an exaggerated, slanted position. The shoe thus sent stress and torque up her leg.

As a word of caution, all athletic-type shoes look pretty good when brand-new. The difference between a $25 pair and a $65 pair is in the materials, construction, and support systems. Remember, you only get what you pay for. Don't buy cheap athletic-type shoes for exercise-walking!

Finally, most people keep their shoes too long. Internal wear and compression are not always obvious. Midsoles compress with the constant loading of the body weight, reducing the cushioning effect. Shoes also stretch sometimes, altering their support. One way to tell if you need new shoes is to have someone watch you walk from behind. If your feet are pronating more in the shoes than when you walk barefoot, get rid of them. Remember that a good pair of walking shoes is not an expense but an investment in your health and happiness.

TAKE CARE OF YOUR FEET

We tend to look down at the tops of our shoes and assume that the foot is a monolithic lump. The foot however, consists of bones, ligaments, and muscles that must interact smoothly and efficiently on every step. Each foot has twenty-six bones, fifty-six ligaments, and thirty-eight muscles. It is a complex piece of biomechanical work. The ability of all those bones, ligaments, and muscles to function naturally and without impediment is essential to the walking gait.

Even though the walking gait is injury-free, many people in this country and other Western industrialized countries experience foot problems when they take up exercise-walking. Some of these problems can be eliminated before they start; others can be managed with the help of a good podiatrist. One of the most common foot problem exercise-walkers—particularly beginning walkers—experience is overuse. The foot of a sedentary person, like the rest of his or her body, is unfit. Many people abruptly start a walking program and activate the foot without gradually getting it into condition by taking short, frequent walks.

The two billion people in less-developed countries who walk barefoot or in sandals use the walking gait as their primary form of locomotion. From their first steps as children to their graves, their feet are used constantly, day in and day out, mile after mile. Their feet become fit and tough and stay that way through their entire lives. Soft, sedentary people in Western industrialized countries spend most of their lives sitting or riding. For many, the foot has lost its strength and durability, much like an arm or leg that has been in a cast.

When I traveled coast to coast doing walking clinics I became aware of the great number of people who have foot problems. Bunions, heel spurs, and hammertoes can make life miserable for a walker. Yet, with the help of a good podiatrist, most of these situations can be managed successfully. My wife, Carol, had both feet operated on for extremely painful bunions ten years ago. Today she walks 3 miles in 39 minutes at 67 years of age.

Managing foot problems sometimes requires an orthotic. An orthotic is a molded bed that slips inside the shoe and gives your foot constant support and balance where it is needed. I know many exercise-walkers who have traveled a lot of happy miles on their orthotics. There are few foot problems that can't be solved, or at least successfully controlled, with today's state-of-the-art podiatry. If you experience nagging foot problems when you take up exercise-walking, I suggest you have a good podiatrist check your feet and walking shoes.

SOCKS

I have on my desk an ad for a major brand of athletic sock that says it is "cushion-engineered." A picture of the sock has arrows pointing to the heel and forefoot, accompanied by this copy, "Heavyweight Plus cushioning across the sole protects the heel and ball against concussion and shock." Utter nonsense! How much concussion and shock can a little bit of yarn on the bottom of your foot absorb?

The role of the sock is to provide an environment between your foot and the shoe. If you have proper shoes, they will take care of all the cushioning you need. Besides, concussion and shock are not a problem for walkers. A smooth-fitting sock that conforms to your foot and doesn't wrinkle is all you need. Wrinkles in a sock will rub your foot and cause blisters. I have acquired more blisters from socks than I have from shoes. Do not buy tube socks. The worst case of blisters I ever had came from a discount store bargain on tube socks—six pairs for six bucks. I began to get blisters under my middle toes. It took me three weeks to figure out that the material of the ill-fitting tube socks was gathering under my toes and rubbing when I toed off. When the exercise-walking movement got big, the sock companies who had been wooing runners saw a larger market and immediately invented "walking socks." But the "engineering" in walking socks is advertising hype.

Cotton socks absorb moisture and lose their shape when wet with sweat. This can cause wrinkles and blisters. There are a number of synthetic materials that wick moisture away from the foot, and I prefer these to cotton or wool. I have been wearing socks made with DuPont Cool Max fiber. However, if the socks you are wearing are not causing you blisters and you are pleased with them, there is no need to change them.

CLOTHING

Walking clothing should be roomy, comfortable, and nonbinding in the legs, arms, and shoulders. Jeans are too restrictive and do not permit the legs enough freedom. Women should not exercise-walk in skirts. Even a wide skirt bumping the front of the leg tends to inhibit a full, fast stride.

I consider my daily walk a workout, and the clothes I wear are the athletic type rather than just an old pair of pants. Buy the new synthetic materials that help wick away the moisture from sweat. Sweats and shorts don't cost much and last a long time. Exercise-walking in workout gear is important for you psychologically because if you dress athletically you'll feel athletic, no matter how old you are. You will walk with greater determination and purpose.

WEATHER: HOT AND COLD

Exercise-walking in hot weather can be treacherous, especially for an older, out-of-shape person. Don't go out in the midday hours if the temperature reaches 90 degrees and above; it can be dangerous. Don't worry about aerobic speed, and cancel your walk if you feel light-headed or dizzy. When we have those July-

August Missouri heat waves, I generally walk at 6 a.m. Even then the combination of heat and humidity makes it difficult to breathe easily. You'll find that such weather makes your legs seem heavy and hard to move; it will test your resolve. As long as you protect yourself against sunstroke and dehydration, however, there is no reason not to walk. You don't have to push as hard or walk as far, but don't give up your routine.

Once in a while in hot, humid weather, I start out slowly and decide to just poke along. By the second mile, when I'm wringing wet with sweat, something seems to break loose, and I finish as strongly as if it were a cool day. Your body will tell you when to go fast and when to coast. Don't assume that you have to hit top speed every day in hot weather, but also don't assume that you can't hit top speed on a hot day. Listen to your body.

Drink plenty of water before you start out and plenty when you come back. Most of us don't drink enough water. Doctors recommend six to eight glasses a day. If you walk aerobically for 30 minutes to an hour each day in hot weather, be sure you drink this much. You'll need it. Also consider taking a water bottle with you, but don't carry it in your hand. It will cause you to have an uneven arm swing. Sports stores and LL Bean sell water bottles that hook on to a belt.

Cold weather is the other extreme to be faced in many parts of the country. As people get older, their tolerance for cold seems to diminish; that's why the Sunbelt is such a popular retirement area. For those of us who don't mind it, cold-weather walking can be the most invigorating and enjoyable of all, but you must dress properly for it. The most dangerous aspect of cold weather for a walker is not low temperature but wind. A wind chill of 10 degrees or lower is something to fear. Even proper clothing can't produce a comfort level at which you can walk with smooth biomechanical movements when it's frigid. Leg muscles take forever to warm up, and on some days they never do.

Weather reports on TV stations announce wind chills in the winter, and in some ways they are more important than actual temperatures. You will find that a light wind of 5 miles per hour and a cold temperature is easier to tolerate and less chilling than a high wind of 20 miles per hour and slightly warmer temperatures.

If you are a cardiac patient, always walk at a temperature range (hot or cold) that your physician thinks is appropriate for you.

On a cold, windy day, the most important rule to remember is *always start your walk headed into the wind*. Doing so is uncomfortable, but it will tell you right away whether it is too cold to walk at all. You won't walk far before you'll know if this is a day when you should just pack it in. If you start out with your back to the wind, you can be a couple of miles from home before you realize that the return trip is unbearable. This happened to me one time and I quickly learned my lesson.

The other negative about wind, particularly gusty wind, is the natural tendency to lean into it, which throws your posture off, and you'll tire your back and shoulder muscles. Even on days when the wind chill is not a factor, wind can louse up your walk because it affects your posture. Cold-weather walking without wind, however, is a delight.

Cold-weather clothing should be worn in layers. It is better to overdress so that you can peel off a layer or two than to be shivering and wishing you had worn more. It is impossible to walk with the proper posture if you are cold, especially if you're feeling the chill in the chest and rib cage. For walking in temperatures below 25 degrees, an essential piece of clothing is a fleece vest. You don't need an expensive goose-down vest; an inexpensive synthetic one works fine. The rest of your clothing can be standard-brand thermal long-john tops and bottoms, turtleneck or mock turtleneck shirts, sweatpants, a light windbreaker, a cap with ear flaps or a stocking cap, and warm gloves or mittens.

Some people have a greater tolerance for cold than others, so you'll have to experiment with how many layers you need at 20, 10, and 0 degrees. Below zero, forget it. Keep your eye on the temperature and wind chill. When in doubt, wear more, not less. Stepping out the front door to test the weather is not a good gauge. You will be tempted to think it is not as cold as it really is because you are still warm, and a few seconds outside won't give you a good indication of what to expect. Put your nylon windbreaker on over your vest; as you heat up, you can peel it off first and tie it around your waist. You are then in a good position to open your vest and let air in around your rib cage if you become really hot. Cold weather helps you burn more calories, which is an added reason to get outside for your walk. It also makes you step right along, and the faster you walk, the warmer you'll feel.

In cold weather many people make the mistake of walking with their hands jammed in the pockets of their jackets. It is important to have your arms loose and swinging freely to counterbalance your leg swing. Insulated gloves or mittens will keep your hands warm. Cold weather invites fast walking, and if your arms are neutralized, your ability to walk fast in a smooth, rhythmic manner is eliminated. You also eliminate the activity of the major muscle groups in the chest, shoulders, and back, which contributes to your caloric expenditure and overall fitness.

RULES OF THE ROAD AND SAFETY TIPS

I walk on two-lane country roads where there are no sidewalks. A cardinal rule for anyone who walks on a road is *always walk facing the traffic*. Other rules of the road are:

- Even though you may have the right-of-way at an intersection, make eye contact with the driver of an approaching car so that he or she will acknowledge your presence.
- Always look both ways before crossing a street or intersection.
- Stay on the outside of a blind curve if the road is narrow.
- On two-lane roads, step onto the shoulder to allow oncoming cars to pass if one is coming from the other direction. It's the courteous and safe thing to do.
- When walking at twilight or at night, always wear reflective strips on your clothing and shoes.
- Wear white or bright-colored clothing on gray, cloudy days. (I wear Day-Glo orange.)

Those of us who live in the serenity of a rural area only have to worry about the dangers of automobiles. Unfortunately, people living in many areas of large cities also have to think about personal safety. Here are some guidelines to follow in that regard:

- Try to find a walking buddy, especially if you are a woman.
- Know the area where you are walking and any businesses that will be open during your walk in case you need to ask them for help. Stay out of isolated areas.
- If possible, walk when there is other pedestrian traffic.

- Don't walk at night in unlit, isolated areas.
- Try to vary your walks so that you don't have a set routine.
- When walking in parks, stay away from dense brush and wooded areas.
- Don't walk close to doorways or courtyards.
- Let someone know where you are going and when you expect to be back.
- Women should consider carrying a police whistle and Mace in their fanny packs.
- Don't wear jewelry. Carry a cell phone if you have one.
- Carry an identification tag in your pocket or fanny pack with your name, address, phone number, and blood type.
- If you are carrying an iPod or wearing headphones, scan the area around you constantly, even glancing backward once in a while. Walk defensively because you may not hear someone coming from the rear.

MALL WALKING

Shopping malls have become a great asset to the exercise-walking movement. Many people walk in them to escape the hazards of city streets, while others like their predictable climate. I have conducted walking clinics in almost a hundred major shopping malls, and many people tell me they wouldn't walk at all if they couldn't do so in a mall.

In the northern tier states, people escape harsh winter weather walking in malls. In the South, particularly in cities like Houston and Miami, which have heat coupled with high humidity, malls provide a comfortable environment. The average age of mall walkers is about 60, so climatic conditions and personal safety are major concerns for them. If you are just starting a walking program and want to walk where the action is, check out a mall near you.

The shopping mall in St. Joseph, Missouri, where I live, is typical of many that cater to "mall walkers." It opens at 6 a.m. to let walkers get an early start. One and a half trips around the perimeter is about a mile. Many of the regular walkers do 3 to 4 miles a day. A few walk at a 15-minute-mile pace, but most of them walk much slower.

Most people at the St. Joseph mall say they are walking for their health and to lose weight. One woman said she has lost 51 pounds by walking. Quite a few people have heart problems. A 68-year-old widower said he likes the opportunity to meet people and has made over a hundred new acquaintances by walking at the mall. There is a certain camaraderie among mall walkers, especially the early birds. The stores don't open until ten o'clock, but all the hard-core walkers are there well before seven.

A shopping mall can be a good place for you to start exercise-walking. You will be exposed to others who have discovered the miracle of walking. You will hear health-improvement and weight-loss stories that will motivate you. Bear in mind that most mall walkers are fighting many of the same problems you have, and you will find it easy to relate to them. Having twenty or thirty people with similar problems giving you encouragement to walk every day may be just what you need to change your lifestyle.

If you decide to walk in a mall, here are a couple of tips. Most people drive to a mall, and women usually bring a purse for their car keys. But carrying a purse or wearing a shoulder bag inhibits free arm swing. Get a small fanny pack to carry your wallet and car keys so that you can walk with vigor and a full arm swing. Also, practically everybody walks every little nook and cranny around the mall's perimeter, which means making too many short turns. This interrupts the pace and rhythm of the walk. Many malls are a quarter of a mile long. Pick the longest straight-away for your walk so that you can sustain a good, strong pace with few turns. A ¼ mile mall, for instance, would permit you to do ½ mile with only one turn. Walk the perimeter for your cool down, when pace is not important. If it is a nice day, try walking the perimeter of the mall's parking lot.

FREQUENTLY ASKED QUESTIONS

My knowledge of walking and exercise is the result of continuous reading and research. From Dr. Lovejoy to Dr. Inman and all the other physicians and experts I have quoted, I have tried to be careful to select only sources that are scientifically correct. By the time you have reached this chapter, you probably have a pretty good idea of how your walking gait came about and how it works biomechanically.

The answers I gave in the question-and-answer parts of my lectures sometimes were my own opinion, but most often they were the result of reading and research. I have covered much about exercise-walking already, but the following are some questions that were asked regularly in my clinics.

Question: What do you think of hand weights and ankle weights?

Answer: Next to an ill-fitting pair of shoes, I can't think of anything that can ruin your walk quicker than hand or ankle weights. Using them is a dumb idea. The recommended use of weights for walkers is kept alive by sources that people assume are reliable. For instance, I have an encyclopedia on wellness, health, and illness prevention that I ordered from one of the finest universities in the United States. I checked the section entitled "Tips and Techniques for a Walking Program." Sure enough, there were those ubiquitous walking weights. The encyclopedia said, "As you get used to walking, carry a six-pound backpack or hand weights. You can substitute a briefcase or shopping bag for the backpack." How would you like to go out for a 3-mile exercise-walk every day carrying a shopping bag or briefcase? How could you swing your arms?

Follow the science and rationale behind my answer, and let common sense be your guide. Why are weights recommended for walkers in the first place? The only reason I can think of is the assumption that they are needed to add *intensity* to the walking gait. But adding weights to walkers to achieve intensity is as outdated as leisure suits. In Chapter 6 you learned to pick up the pace of your walk simply by swinging your arms faster with the bent-arm technique and by teaching your leg muscles to fire faster. The assumption that exercise-walking lacks the intensity to be aerobic is without merit.

Weights aren't added to cyclists; they are told to pedal faster if they want exercise intensity. Weights aren't added to cross-country skiers; they just ski faster. You never see knowledgeable runners carrying weights. Everyone assumes that these exercises are intensive enough to be aerobic, but so is exercise-walking if it is done properly.

Many reading this book are taking up walking for weight control, and the companies who sell weights often make outrageous and unfounded claims about how many extra calories they will help you burn. An issue of the *Tufts University Diet and Nutrition Letter* cited a caloric expenditure study involving walkers with weights. It reported, "When eleven overweight people at the University of Missouri walked briskly with one-pound hand weights for a full thirty minutes, they burned only about 12 more calories than they did without weights—a couple of Lifesavers worth."

Dr. Harvey B. Simon, assistant professor of medicine at Harvard Medical School, gave some additional unimpressive caloric numbers in the September-October 1989 issue of *The Walking Magazine*: "A 135 pound woman who walks vigorously can expect to burn about 200 calories in thirty minutes. Add 10 pounds of weights and you can expect to burn about 10 calories more. . . . You would have to carry those weights for about 300 miles to drop just one extra pound because of [them]. For comparison, walking itself will have taken off 30 pounds by then."

Walking should be a smooth, fluid, natural exercise. Biomechanically your arms and legs are properly balanced and should swing freely. Any weight you add to the ankles or hands unbalances your limbs and alters their normal swing for the worse, possibly even to the point of causing injury. Ankle weights can hyperextend your knees, and weights in general ruin your walk. Your object is to get the arm and leg pendulums swinging faster, and you can't do so by adding weights. On a risk-reward basis there are few things a walker could do that would be more counterproductive.

Question: I live where there are hills. Will I burn a lot more calories walking uphill?

Answer: A few nice, rolling hills add variety to a walk and may or may not burn a few extra calories. I often read articles in which a walker is advised that he or she can burn more calories by walking up hills. That's true, but the writers blithely seem to assume that there is one continuous hill. How about the return downhill? Without getting into a deep technical explanation of "positive work" and "negative work," you already know that it is easier to walk down a hill or downstairs than it is to walk up. Gravity is pulling against you going up and pulling you toward your line of travel going down. Up is positive work, and down is negative work. That's a bit oversimplified, but you get the point.

If you walk up a hill, you have to walk down the other side, which burns fewer calories than walking up or walking on the level. When I wear a heart-rate monitor, it is interesting to observe how quickly my heart rate goes up when I'm climbing a hill, even though my pace slows, and how quickly it starts to drop as I crest the hill and head down the other side. I have to increase my speed considerably to keep my heart rate up when walking downhill, and so will you. If you average the up-and-down caloric expenditure of walking up hills, it may not be much better than that of a fast, sustainable pace on level ground.

Question: Is there a particular way to walk uphill or downhill?

Answer: Going uphill, one's first inclination is to bend at the waist and lean into the hill. That's wrong, and if you do so, you will soon have lower-back muscles that are fatigued and hurting. Leonard Jansen, the former race-walking analyst at the United States Olympic Training Center, advises that you should maintain proper erect posture and *shorten your stride* walking up a hill (see Figure 9.5).

Your pace will slow but the pull of gravity as you go uphill will make you work harder, and your heart rate will actually increase. Remember that, when you walk up stairs, the average stair riser is only about 8 inches high, so your step is automatically shortened. Keep your head up, your back straight from your ears to your ankles, and your shoulders over your hips.

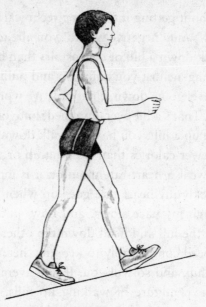

FIGURE 9.5

You can lean forward slightly by bending at the ankles, as race-walkers do, but don't lose your posture. If the hill is extremely steep, like some of those in San Francisco, forget speed altogether and walk up it with the best posture possible. Hills like that create more posture problems than they are worth and are not enjoyable for exercise-walking. I recommend that you find a level place to walk if you live in a very hilly area.

Walking downhill presents a different challenge. It is easy to keep your posture, but how do you increase speed to keep your heart rate up without jarring yourself senseless? Keep your body erect, almost as if you are leaning backward, away from the slope of the hill. This is a good way to practice erect posture, and it is easy to hold your head up. With your bent arms pumping fast to keep up with your accelerated leg swing, let gravity help pull you down the hill as fast as you can make your legs and feet move in a smooth, coordinated manner. This position also gives you a shorter leg swing, so that your foot doesn't have as far to drop down the hill at heel plant, and this reduces the jarring effect of downhill walking.

Question: *When is the best time to walk—morning or evening?*

Answer: The best time is any time you can walk *consistently*. Your body doesn't care whether it is morning, noon, or night. We have two active dogs and they are anxious to go at 6:30 a.m., seven days a week. That is when we walk. You and your schedule should determine when you walk. Some folks are natural morning people and jump out of bed raring to go. If you are one of those, get up early enough to get a good walk in, shower, have a nutritious breakfast, and when you head for work you will be set for a high-energy day.

Another good time for walking is an hour or two before dinner. Walking then reduces your appetite and gives you an exercise-induced caloric afterburn that helps dispose of the evening meal's calories. If you have a stressful job, there isn't any better way than a brisk or aerobic walk to clear your mind and work off frustrations or hostilities that may have accumulated during the day. A vigorous walk after work will energize you physically and soothe you mentally. The often prescribed tranquilizers cannot do for you what a long, hard walk will do.

Question: *I live in an area where there is a lot of traffic pollution and smog. Are there better times than others to exercise, and how does this affect me?*

Answer: Unfortunately, millions of exercisers live in high-density cities with traffic pollution and/or smog. They should try to walk early in the morning, before the pollution reaches its maximum concentrations.

According to Dr. Bryant Stamford, Professor and Chair of the Department of Exercise Science at Hanover College, carbon monoxide and ozone present the biggest threats to exercisers. Exhaust fumes from automobiles are the major contributor to carbon-monoxide pollution. Ozone results from the sun acting on nitrogen dioxide and certain hydrocarbons; it is a predominant component of city smog. In his "Exercise Adviser" column for *The Physician and Sportsmedicine Magazine,* he stated: "Exercising in heavy traffic places an added strain on the heart, which must work harder to counteract the increased intake of carbon monoxide and decreased oxygen concentration." Dr. Stamford suggested six ways city exercisers can minimize the risks of encountering air pollution:

- Avoid exercising during peak traffic hours.
- Avoid exercising when the sun is brightest; ozone levels increase on sunny days.
- Respect air-pollution alerts and exercise accordingly.
- Exercise in open areas, where air currents can move about freely, dispersing pollutants.
- Be aware of exercising or resting for prolonged periods under shade trees; they can trap pollutants.
- Avoid ambient cigarette smoke before and after exercise. If you are a smoker, never smoke just after exercise; wait until you are breathing normally. Quitting smoking is even better.

Question: *Is it better to exercise before or after a meal?*
Answer: It is best to exercise an hour or two before, or at least two hours after, eating your meal. I like to exercise before

eating and I have some of my best and fastest walks when I feel hungry. Vigorous exercise tends to blunt the appetite. When you work up a good sweat in warm weather, you will come in very thirsty but not very hungry. That's when you will drink a lot of fluids (preferably water) and tend to eat less, which helps with weight control.

Exercising vigorously right after a meal is ill-advised. In his "Exercise Adviser" column, Dr. Stamford cautioned: "During vigorous exercise the blood is withdrawn from the abdomen and shunted toward the working muscles. Digestion is put on hold, which can cause considerable distress." Instead of flopping down in front of the TV and letting your eyes glaze over after dinner, take a slow, easy stroll. In the parts of the country that have four distinct seasons, spring, summer, and fall are great strolling months.

A stroll after dinner has another significant benefit: marital communication. Get away from the TV and telephone. Spend 20 or 30 minutes reestablishing your ability to communicate with each other while strolling along. A walk after dinner is the catalyst for sharing problems and finding solutions. In this hectic world, it might strengthen some frayed marriage bonds.

Question: Should I breathe in any particular way while walking?

Answer: Walking at a slow pace doesn't put any demands on breathing except for extremely overweight people. As you pick up your pace, however, particularly if you move on to aerobic walking, your method of breathing can affect performance. There is a tendency to breathe shallowly, which only supplies air to the upper passages—the mouth, throat, and bronchi. These areas do not participate in the oxygen-gas exchange with the blood. The lungs are where oxygen is transferred to the bloodstream so that it can be pumped out to the muscles by the heart.

As you walk faster and need more oxygen, breathe deeply. Inhale to capacity by expanding your stomach as you fill up your lungs. Some race-walking coaches call this *belly breathing*. Many people try to fill their lungs by sucking in their stomachs as they inhale. To try it both ways, stand up and draw in as much air as possible by expanding your stomach. Let the air out; then draw in as much air as possible by sucking in your stomach. Do you feel the difference? If you fill your lungs several times each way, you'll find that your lungs fill all the way to the top if you expand your stomach. Develop your own comfortable relationship between breathing and stride frequency. Breathe as you need, and breathe deeply. Correct posture with a straight back opens up the rib cage so that your lungs can fill to capacity.

Question: When I walk real fast, I sometimes get a sharp pain in my side. What is it and what can I do about it?

Answer: This is the puzzling side stitch, which seems to defy diagnosis. There are several theories about it, but no clear consensus. The American Fitness Association book *Conquering Athletic Injuries* states: "Because the mechanism of the side-stitch is poorly understood, there is no standard treatment." The baffling thing about side stitches is that they intermittently attack some exercisers but never others.

There are a few consistent clues, however. Side stitches seem to appear more often in exercisers who are building fitness level than in fully conditioned athletes. They occur near the bottom of the rib cage when the exerciser is at an intense level of exercise, and they usually fade when the intensity drops. I remember getting side stitches off and on when I was building up my fitness. They always went away when I reduced my pace. Side stitches are an uncomfortable annoyance but nothing to worry about. They will probably disappear once you have reached a good fitness level. In the meantime, when one occurs, slow down.

Question: I sweat a lot when I walk fast in warm weather. How much water should I drink, and do I need any of those special athletic drinks?

Answer: Unless you are walking for more than an hour or live in a hot climate, the normal recommended intake of six to eight glasses of water a day should be enough. The problem is that very few people—including me—actually drink eight full glasses of water every day. But I know I should, and so should you.

Water makes up about 60 percent of the body weight and is used in a number of body functions, such as digestion, absorption, circulation, excretion, nutrient transmission, tissue maintenance, and temperature regulation. Besides sweat, you lose water from the body in urine, feces, and when you exhale. Drinking lots of water year round, not merely when you sweat, is a healthful thing to do.

Some of your daily water requirements can come from juices, fruits, and vegetables that have a high water content, as well as caffeine-free soft drinks. Coffee and tea (regular), caffeinated soft drinks, and alcohol do not count as water intake. Alcohol causes dehydration, and the other drinks are diuretics that actually make you lose fluid.

Sports drinks such as Gatorade, which you see along the sidelines at football games and sporting events, are expensive relative to water and unnecessary for the average exerciser. They are sometimes called electrolyte replacement drinks because they contain sodium and potassium, which help balance the acidity-alkalinity of fluids in the body cells. But the *University of California at Berkeley Wellness Letter* pointed out that "most sports drinks actually contain far less potassium than a glass of orange juice." It added: "There is rarely any need to replace electrolytes by consuming special 'sport drinks' or mineral supplements. These minerals are lost in small quantities that can easily be replaced by a normal diet." Further, "The sugar content in most of these drinks is excessive." All things considered, it's hard to beat plain water. There are a lot of bottled waters on the market, and some of them are not as safe as, or any better than, tap water from a well-regulated municipal source. In some cities, however, the water may taste a little odd, so people buy bottled water. At times I want to drink something fizzy, and plain water doesn't fill the bill. I keep several bottles of plain sparkling water in the refrigerator which is nothing more than purified, carbonated water. It has no sodium added, like club soda, which may contain 30 to 65 milligrams of sodium per 8 ounces. Squeeze some lime or lemon in sparkling water or put about a third of a glass of orange juice in it for your own inexpensive, healthful, homemade "sports drink."

Question: How much should I warm up and cool down?

Answer: A low-intensity stroll at a 20-minute-mile pace or slower doesn't require any warm-up. Simply start walking, find your comfort zone, and continue. The moderate-intensity brisk walker will probably find that a 17- to 19-minute-mile pace feels best for the first ¼ to ½ mile before moving up to the full brisk pace. The high-intensity aerobic walker will be more fit and can easily handle a 15-minute-mile pace from the start for a warm-up pace, gradually increasing speed after the first ½ mile.

Fast walkers generally agree that their first mile is their most sluggish. It takes almost a mile before the leg muscles really get warmed up, loose, and rhythmic. After a mile, aerobic walkers, and even brisk walkers, will find another level of speed that seems more effortless. On my 3-mile walks, my third mile is the smoothest and fastest, and it seems to require less effort than the first. If you start at a faster pace than I have suggested, you won't injure yourself, but you probably will find that the first mile requires more effort than the rest of your walk.

The cool-down for a walker is less of a problem than for a runner. Strollers don't really have any cooling down to do, but they should stretch at the end of their walk—as should all walkers. On a hot day, brisk walkers may want to stroll for a couple of hundred yards to cool down. Aerobic walkers should drop their arms from the bent-arm swing and stroll for 5 or 10 minutes to let their heart rates drop.

If you have had a hard workout and have an elevated heart rate, Dr. T. L. Mitchell of the Cooper Clinic advises that *your heart rate should drop at least 12 beats in the first minute you stop exercising.* If your heart rate remains elevated, you could be exercising at a level for which you are not conditioned or you could have some underlying health problem. Older exercisers in particular should be aware of the latter. Dr. Mitchell believes it would be wise to consult with your physician if this occurs. This is another reason I believe heart rate monitors are a good investment.

Question: What do you think of pedometers?

Answer: My experience with pedometers has not been good. I have had several given to me as gifts. When I checked them against an accurate measured mile, some registered a longer distance by as much as $\frac{2}{10}$ of a mile. The September 2005 *Tufts Uni-*

versity Health and Nutrition Letter quoted a study that tested 13 brands of pedometers for accuracy and found that some over- or underestimated steps by 20 to 40 percent. You definitely want more accuracy than that. I am a stickler for distance accuracy, because I time a lot of my walks. I bought a Measure Master wheel made by the Rolatape Corporation (800-435-1859 or www.rolatape.com) and they are accurate down to 1/10 of a foot. I have my 3-mile course marked every 1/4 mile by a small spray-painted Day-Glo orange dot near the bottom of a fence post or tree, or at the side of the road.

If you have a walking club or a neighborhood group that walks a set course, or several courses, it is better for the group to buy one of these measuring wheels than for several people to buy pedometers, which would cost more and not be as accurate.

Question: What about walking to music—does it help?

Answer: I think walking to music helps in every way. Next to a good pair of walking shoes I believe an iPod (or its technical equivalent) is one of the best long-term investments an exercise-walker can make. I have often referred to the *rhythm* of walking, and nothing helps this better than music. Many women tell me that walking to music makes them walk not only more but faster.

Walkers moving beyond the brisk pace to the 12-minute-mile aerobic pace will definitely become looser and more fluid if they have a good music beat to drive them. Music reduces the mechanical action of the walking gait by increasing the rhythmic flow of the walker. Even slower walkers find their exercise time passes more quickly with the soothing, entertaining beat of their favorite music. When walking to music be aware that you may not be able to hear cars coming from behind. Do not become musically preoccupied and forget to check carefully for oncoming vehicles at intersections.

My most important advice to anyone who uses an iPod is *never, ever carry it in your hand*. This is a major mistake made by many people. Although the iPod is light, subconsciously it will cause you to alter your arm swing. A properly balanced arm swing is essential for all walkers, but especially for brisk and aerobic walkers. Carry your iPod in a small fanny pack so that your hands are unencumbered and your arms get a complete swing cycle.

I grew up with the big-band sounds of Glenn Miller, Tommy Dorsey, and Harry James, and on many of my walks I get immersed in the nostalgia of my youth. These are some of my best walks. Each generation has its own music and the special memories associated with it. Take your music with you on your walk, and you will cruise along smoother, faster, and happier than you ever thought possible. As the current generation says, "Rock on!"

TEN

High-intensity Walking
The Undiscovered Cross-training Exercise

THE OXYGEN INTAKE CLUE

In the spring of 1985, when I was researching my first book, *Aerobic Walking,* I found a graph (Figure 10.1) that showed the relationship of oxygen intake to the velocity of walking and running in internationally ranked race-walkers. The numbers across the bottom of the chart indicate the walker's speed in kilometers per hour. (Since kilometers are not widely used in the United States and are unfamiliar to most, a key number to remember is 8 kilometers per hour equals 5 miles per hour, which is the equivalent of 12-minute miles). I added the circle to the graph to

FIGURE 10.1

RELATIONSHIPS BETWEEN OXYGEN CONSUMPTION AND VELOCITY FOR
WALKING AND RUNNING ON A TREADMILL IN COMPETITION WALKERS

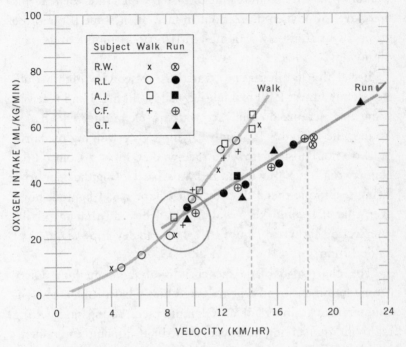

Source: D.R. Menier and L.G.C.E. Pugh, "The relation of oxygen intake and velocity of walking and
running in competition walkers," J.Physiol. 197:717, 168.

focus your attention on the point where the lines of oxygen utilization between walking and running cross, which is about 8
kilometers per hour. This is called a metabolic intersection,
where the energy costs of two activities meet.

Notice that from about a 12-minute mile on, a walker uses
considerably more oxygen than a runner if both maintain the
same speed. I find most people don't believe this or understand

this proven fact. Even though an exercise-walker could not achieve the top speeds of these race-walkers, many aerobic walkers walk a 12-minute mile or faster, which puts them at this high level of oxygen utilization. In fact, at the time I found the graph I was routinely walking at a 10- or 11-minute-mile pace on my daily walks.

It was this graph that motivated me to see how high I could elevate my fitness level by high-intensity walking. I had received some instructions on the race-walking technique from Larry Young, the United States' only Olympic race-walking medalist, but I do not consider myself a race-walker. I just get out on the country roads near my home and walk hard, using the bent-arm-swing technique that I described in Chapter 6. I figured, however, that if I could keep walking well beyond that metabolic intersection shown in Figure 10.1, I should develop the fitness of a good runner.

The chart also made me curious about something Larry Young had mentioned when I asked him what problems he encountered in training for an Olympic race. Young said getting highly fit and staying fresh was sometimes difficult. He remembered that, when he tended to get stale in the late stages of heavy training, he would occasionally *run* the last 5 miles of a 10-mile workout at about an 8-minute-mile pace to relax his mind and his legs. Young said running was less intense mentally and physically than walking at that pace, and it seemed to freshen him up. I asked him if he could have run much faster than an 8-minute-mile pace, and he said he was sure he could, but speed was not his reason for running.

This aroused my interest. How could an athlete training for a specific event unrelated to running run 5 miles in 40 minutes literally on a whim—in fact, do it because it seemed relatively effortless? I felt sure a swimmer, cyclist, or rower could not do that. This was a glaring exception to the specificity principle; I did not believe distance runners who ran at a 5-minute-mile pace, for instance, could switch to walking at a 9-minute-mile pace without cross-training. This was unique, that a high-intensity walker could transfer his or her aerobic capacity to running when the running gait does not possess a similar reciprocity with walking.

I drew the dotted lines down in Figure 10.1 to the kilometers-per-hour line from the fastest walking speed and the fastest running speed. It showed that those competitive walkers had walked at a pace of about 6.6-minute miles but also ran at speeds up to 5.4-minute miles. If they weren't cross-trained in running, how could they do that? How could they achieve a higher oxygen intake walking than running? Isn't running supposed to require more oxygen for a higher aerobic capacity than walking?

The study clearly showed that these competitive walkers were capable of developing oxygen intakes comparable to those of many competitive runners. There seemed to be another subtlety in the study. These walkers were also able to develop running velocities (5.4-minute pace) similar to those of distance runners, apparently without cross-training. I say apparently because at that time I had no way of proving they hadn't cross-trained. I could only assume it. If my assumption was correct, the possibilities of using high-intensity walking for aerobic athletic conditioning and training seemed endless. I believed duplicating this study with competitive walkers who were definitely not cross-trained was imperative to resolve the question.

THE HIGH-INTENSITY WALKING STUDY

The expanded role high-intensity walking could play in athletic training would call for a specifically designed high-performance walking shoe. The Brown Shoe Company was interested in the sales potential and provided the funding for the study. My search for a top exercise physiologist with research experience to conduct the study led me to Dr. William Byrnes of the Department of Kinesiology at the University of Colorado, Boulder. He checked the scientific literature and found that no one had ever tested for such a cross-training effect. Dr. Byrnes enlisted his friend and former college mentor, Dr. Jay T. Kearney, who at the time was the head of Sports Science at the United States Olympic Training Center (USOTC) in Colorado Springs, to assist in the protocol design and testing.

The study that resulted in Figure 10.1 was conducted in 1968 by D. R. Menier and L.G.C.E. Pugh in the Pyrenees Mountains at a French Olympic training center. The four competitive walkers in the study were in training for the 1968 Olympics. Larry Young won his first Olympic medal (bronze) in the 50K race-walk at Mexico City in 1968, and he raced against the French walkers in the study. He later confirmed to me that his opponents were *not* cross-trained in running. Young said that most race-walkers of that period thought running would be counterproductive to their training regimen, and they worked solely on walking speed and technique. Additionally, the term *cross-training* had not even become part of exercise nomenclature in 1968.

Dr. Byrnes's protocol had a clever wrinkle. He felt our study would be more comprehensive if he tested walkers *and* runners who were not cross-trained in the opposite gait. He could then measure the aerobic transferability in both directions. To establish a standard level of athletic competence for the athletes to be tested, he and Dr. Kearney decided to test only competitive walkers who were capable of walking at an 8-minute-mile pace or better for 10 kilometers (6.2 miles). The runners had to be capable of running at a 6-minute-mile pace or better for 10 kilometers. They wanted nationally ranked athletes.

The actual protocol was quite extensive and complex. In simple lay language, however, it boiled down to this. Each participant had to walk on a motorized treadmill at predetermined progressive speeds to reach a heart rate of 170. At that point, the treadmill grade was increased by 2.5 percent every 2 minutes until the subject reached volitional exhaustion. On a separate day the participants would repeat a similar process using the running gait.

For the simplicity of recruiting top athletes and conducting the tests in the most convenient location, it was decided to conduct the physical aspects of the study at USOTC. This decision led to an unexpected plus: the Mexican National Race-walking Team came to USOTC in September for physiological testing on their sophisticated equipment, and Dr. Kearney persuaded them to participate in our study.

This was a real coup. The Mexicans were some of the best walkers in the world. Dr. Byrnes was enthused because he would be able to test world-class athletes with exceptional aerobic capacities. He and Dr. Kearney had tested the U.S. men's race-walking team in August, and the U.S. women's team was to be tested in November.

To my disappointment, my travel schedule did not permit me to observe the U.S. men's or the Mexicans' tests. I was able to attend the women's test, however. Five of the six women walkers who were tested were on the U.S. race-walking team. When I walked into USOTC the day of the test, three of our walkers—Lynn Weik, the American road record holder for the 15K and 20K; Teresa Vaill, 1990 and 1991 indoor 3K champion; and Susan Liers, who held several American records in the 1970s—were stretching in preparation for the treadmills. I watched those young women walk to exhaustion one day and run to exhaustion the next. It was an athletic endurance contest. As each one neared volitional exhaustion, her fellow walkers, Dr. Kearney, Dr. Byrnes, and I joined in to root them on. This was a very tough protocol.

From the time the study started, I questioned Dr. Byrnes about when he would test some nationally ranked runners. Drs. Kearney and Byrnes begged, pleaded, coaxed, and cajoled many runners and running teams of the competency level they needed to participate in the two treadmill tests. A few agreed to do the running test, but *none* would do the walking. All participants of the study had to be unpaid volunteers, and all of the race-walkers had willingly volunteered.

It was unthinkable, in my view, that someone of Dr. Kearney's importance and stature at the Olympic level could not persuade a few runners to take a treadmill test for a protocol designed to demonstrate an aerobic cross-training effect that could be used by *all* athletes. The great irony of this is that if the aerobic transferability premise was proven, training regimens for runners could be altered to incorporate some high-intensity walking. This would probably reduce running injuries and prolong running careers. Runners would benefit far more than walkers. Dr. Byrnes quickly calmed my fears that the study would be flawed without the runners. He pointed out that the main thrust of the study was to see if high-intensity walking could produce a similar oxygen intake in the running gait without cross-training. For that we needed walkers—which we had. The runners were not critical to the integrity of the study.

BINGO!

The study abstract and the many charts that were the result of the testing were presented on April 19, 1991, by Drs. Byrnes and Kearney, at the International Congress on Sports Medicine and Human Performance in Vancouver.

The abstract for the study begins: "Fifteen national team race walkers (RW) (9 males and 6 females) from the United States (US) and ten national RW (5 males and 5 females) from Mexico (Mex) agreed to participate in a series of physiological tests." Then followed all the statistical data and procedural explanations. It was the last sentence of the abstract that made me shout, "Bingo!" It said, "*These athletes are capable of achieving similar VO$_2$ max values for race walking and running, which indicates a potential cross-training effect.*" (Emphasis added.) I kept reading that sentence over and over. It threw open the door for high-intensity walking to be utilized as a new approach to athletic training.

Dr. Byrnes posted a graph (Figure 10.2) that illustrated the average race-walking and running maximal oxygen uptakes for U.S. and Mexican national team members. It clearly shows that all these athletes were able to achieve similar VO$_2$ max values in both the running and walking gaits without cross-training.

For the average person reading this book, the term *maximal oxygen uptake* doesn't have much meaning. It is an important measurement, however, used by exercise physiologists to determine the limit of oxygen utilization attainable by an athlete (or

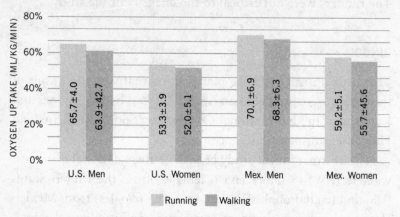

FIGURE 10.2
RACEWALKING AND RUNNING MAXIMAL OXYGEN UPTAKES
FOR UNITED STATES AND MEXICAN NATIONAL TEAM MEMBERS

Source: U.S. Olympic Training Center Study, funded by Brown Shoe Co.

individual) based on his or her level of aerobic fitness. The Menier and Pugh study used the term *oxygen intake,* which means the same thing.

The highest average numbers ever achieved in oxygen uptake were by some very elite, highly trained cross-country skiers who were able to reach the mid-80s. According to Dr. Kearney, a "handful of elite runners may hit the low 80s," but most elite runners will test in the upper 70s. Very good nationally ranked runners will test in the low 70s or upper 60s. The averages shown here are excellent because they were achieved in *both* the walking and running gaits without the benefit of cross-training. One male Mexican walker actually had an oxygen uptake of 77 walking and 78 running. That is a phenomenal performance, and, as Dr. Kearney said several times, "Those Mexicans have big engines!"

By "big engines" he meant their hearts. The Mexican men's
hearts in particular had enormous capacities to pump huge volumes of blood at relatively few beats per minute for the work
they were doing. Figure 10.3 shows the Mexican men's "engines" compared with the Americans' during the walking part of
the protocol. At every measured velocity across the bottom of
the chart, their hearts were beating considerably *less* than the
American men's. This indicates that the Mexicans in the study

FIGURE 10.3

A COMPARISON OF THE HEART RATE RESPONSES DURING RACEWALKING
FOR THE MALE MEMBERS OF THE UNITED STATES AND MEXICAN
NATIONAL TEAMS BETWEEN 7.0 AND 8.5 MPH

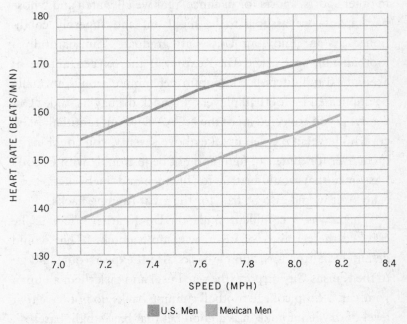

Source: U.S. Olympic Training Center Study, funded by Brown Shoe Co.

could carry their speed over a great distance with less fatigue. In other words, they would likely win the race.

There is an interesting parallel between this study and the one in 1968. Menier and Pugh made a specific notation that an internationally ranked marathon runner serving as a control in their study "had a VO_2 max of 70 ml/kg/min—a surprisingly high value considering the altitude" (see check mark on the right-hand side in Figure 10.1). That study was conducted at 5,940 feet. The elevation of Colorado Springs is 6,035 feet, so the oxygen uptakes generated in that rarefied atmosphere by all of the walkers are indeed impressive.

As I studied the graph, I was groping for a way to explain to readers of this book how those numbers might relate to athletes in other sports, sports for instance, that we all watch and whose participants we assume to be highly fit and superbly conditioned. As an Ohio State University graduate, I am naturally a football fan, so I asked Dr. Kearney if the oxygen uptake of around 70 milliliters per kilogram per minute would normally be duplicated by football players. In mock dismay he said, "Oh, Casey! If you collected *all* of the NCAA Division I football players who have an oxygen uptake above seventy, you could invite them over for dinner tonight and not be in trouble with Carol." I assumed that would be true for linemen and linebackers, but I asked if it would also be true for the great running backs.

There was a confident smile on Dr. Kearney's face as he cranked the certainty of his answer up a notch. "That would definitely be true for running backs also. I expect you could go to the Kansas City airport (the one I use) and pick them all up in your car." If top college football running backs do not have that level of oxygen uptake, it is a good bet that basketball, baseball, tennis, or hockey players wouldn't either.

The walking gait has been considered a "moderate activity" and has not been tested at high-intensity levels. Although the 1968 study by Menier and Pugh established a high oxygen uptake for Olympic-level race walkers, no one picked up on the fact that these athletes actually had a *double-gaited fitness* and could transfer their walking fitness to the running gait. The study by Drs. Byrnes and Kearney clearly demonstrated again that an Olympic-caliber race-walker can transfer a high aerobic fitness level to running without cross-training.

The only question remaining is whether high-intensity walking performed at levels considerably *less* than Olympic-caliber race walking would have a trickle-down effect. Would it produce the fitness and aerobic capacity maintained by NCAA Division I football players, NFL football players, and participants in other sports? I am confident it would.

MY PERSONAL EXPERIMENT

There was one nagging loose end about all of this still in the back of my mind that had to be resolved. I wanted to know if I could transfer *my* fitness level from walking back to running. I had procrastinated for several years on trying to find out because I feared doing irreparable harm to my fragile right knee.

In early 1984, the combination of running and arthritis finally took its toll, and my orthopedic doctor said, "Your running days are over!" I had not run ten steps since. On November 1, 1990, at my annual physical at the Cooper Clinic, I tested superior on the treadmill for a 50-year-old and excellent for a 30-year-old and younger (I was 62). Not as good as my 1985 treadmill test, but I had reduced my walking frequency, duration, and intensity after an arthroscopic knee operation in 1987. This prolonged the time until 1995, when I had to have an artificial replacement for my arthritic right knee.

The day after my physical, I decided it was time to see if I could run as fast or faster than I walk. I was in excellent physical condition, but the thought of running on my arthritic knee had all the appeal of a root canal. I dreaded doing it, but I knew I would never have peace of mind until I did. I believed so strongly in the premise of walking's aerobic transferability to running that I wanted to experience it personally. To me, it was the difference between reading about an earthquake and being there while the ground shakes under my feet.

I started walking down my 2-mile flat course and decided I would walk the first mile at a comfortable 12-minute-mile pace to warm up. It was a delightfully cool morning with just the hint of a breeze. The conditions were perfect. At the ½-mile mark I was pretty well warmed up and walking effortlessly at a shade less than a 12-minute-mile pace when a moment of indecision hit me. Here I was within fifty days of my sixty-third birthday, in perfect health, financially secure, enjoying life, and I was about to ignore strong warnings from my doctor.

My commitment was irreversible, however; I wavered only for a moment. At the 1-mile mark I hit my stopwatch and apprehensively started to run for the first time in *six years*. If my knee held up, I had decided, I would run 2 miles at an easy loping pace. Eight- to 9-minute miles had been my regular pace during my running days.

The first couple of hundred yards seemed strange and fairly effortless, but I quickly realized I didn't have a sense of a running pace anymore. I couldn't tell if I was in a slow jog or running at a respectable speed. I also noticed that I was running with a slight limp. My knee wasn't actually hurting, but I was expecting it to, so I was consciously favoring my right leg. I was running unbalanced, which I knew would contribute to unnecessary fatigue in my good leg, so I got back on an even keel with both legs—for a while.

After a half mile, I was breathing a bit more heavily than when I am in a 10-minute-mile aerobic walk, but I wasn't short of breath and knew I could go faster if I wanted to. At the ¾-mile mark, I was curious about what my pace was and anxious to finish the first mile. As I hit the orange mile mark I have at the side of the road, I glanced at my stopwatch. It registered 8 minutes, 52 seconds. Piece of cake! I turned and headed back for the second mile.

At the ¼-mile mark, I was starting to feel some pain in the right knee. It wasn't imaginary this time, but it didn't become constant until I had passed the ½-mile mark. By then I was consciously running with a limp but determined to finish. When I hit the mile mark, my stopwatch registered 18 minutes and 6 seconds for the 2 miles. My knee felt as if it were on fire in deep on the medial side, where the cartilage is gone, but I was smiling anyhow. I knew I could have gone faster if the knee had been sound.

The results of the study at USOTC were yet to come, but at that moment my *personal* study had proven my point. Although the scientific community calls what I did "anecdotal," I knew what I did had to be grounded in the walking gait's unique aberration in the specificity principle. It was not an accidental fluke that at almost 63 years of age and not having run in over six years I could run 2 miles at a 9-minute-mile average. You can't fake that.

Once the momentary euphoria of my accomplishment wore off, I became quite aware of my painful right knee. The 5-minute ride home seemed twice as long as normal. When I hit the house, I downed two aspirin, took a hot shower, and had an ice pack on the knee, all in the space of a few minutes. The rest of the day was spent on the couch with an ice pack. By evening the pain had settled down, and there was no swelling. I took two aspirin at bedtime and had a deep sleep of satisfaction. The next morning the knee was a little tender, but after two days of rest I was back out walking with no pain. I had my personal moment of truth and had felt the ground shake.

The study at the USOTC probably sheds less light on how high-intensity walking can be converted to a universal form of athletic conditioning than what I did on Riverside Road that November day. The Olympic-class race-walkers demonstrated that very high oxygen uptakes can be achieved with very high-intensity walking and then transferred to the running gait without cross-training. However, they did it at a walking speed unattainable by most other athletes. That's the bad news. The good news is that other athletes don't need those kinds of oxygen uptakes for their athletic conditioning. Only other race-walkers, middle- and long-distance runners, and cross-country skiers need oxygen capacity in those ranges. I was able to demonstrate the trickle-down effect of aerobic transferability. My walking intensity in the 10- to 12-minute-mile range was convertible to a 9-minute-mile running pace at the age of 63—and with an arthritic knee. Imagine what kind of double-gaited aerobic conditioning a young male or female athlete with two good legs could achieve with high-intensity walking.

CROSS-TRAINING WITH WALKING ENDORSED BY RUNNING ICON

No one hungers more for validity than the solitary contrarian trying to scale a wall of conventional wisdom. Scientific giants such as Copernicus and Galileo experienced that hunger when they reasoned that the earth revolves around the sun. Intellectuals and scholars at the great universities of their time rejected such unconventional thinking.

In my pursuit to establish walking as a viable cross-training exercise for running and other physical activities that require an elevated aerobic capacity, I had yearned for someone who shared my vision. Not just anyone, but someone who commanded the respect of the exercise community. My yearning was fulfilled beyond all expectations in the September 1990 issue of *The Physician and Sportsmedicine* magazine in Dr. George Sheehan's column, titled "Walking: Underrated Training Aid." Dr. Sheehan speculated on all of my premises about using walking as an athletic training aid and even opened up possibilities I had overlooked.

Many readers of this book may not have heard of the late Dr. Sheehan, but anyone who was a serious runner during the eighties and early nineties certainly would have. He was considered the patriarch of the running movement. The permanent title for his monthly column in *The Physician and Sportsmedicine* magazine was "Running Wild." Dr. Sheehan was also the medical editor for *Runner's World* magazine and the author of many books related to running, including *Medical Advice for Runners* and *Running and Being*. Dr. Sheehan was in his early seventies and retired from his medical practice after almost forty years as a cardiologist.

At major running events and physical fitness meetings, Dr. Sheehan was sought after as a speaker. Among hard-core runners, he commanded respect bordering on adulation. No one had a better insight into the runners' mentality and how they viewed walkers. In his later years, Dr. Sheehan occasionally walked as a substitute for his usual runs and freely admitted that while walking, "I come up with as many good ideas as I do on a run."

As a keen observer of his fellow runners, Sheehan noticed their disdain for walkers during one of his walks. He wrote, "I saw a runner friend approaching me. I raised my hand in greeting but he ran right by without recognizing me." Sheehan now takes note of runners passing when he walks, and rarely do they give him a glance. "Yet if I were running, I know I would get a friendly word, or at least a wave," he said.

I had long suspected that most runners viewed walking with contempt, but I wasn't aware of the depth of that contempt until Dr. Sheehan wrote in his September 1990 column: "Walkers and walking are of no interest to runners. They regard walking as an entry-level exercise practiced by non-athletes, a low-intensity, noncompetitive pursuit that has no place in the exciting world of road racing. . . . I think most runners have the idea that walking has nothing to offer them relative to training for their sport." I am sure he didn't know how prescient this comment was. Almost ninety days to the day after I read Dr. Sheehan's column, Dr. Byrnes informed me that he and Dr. Kearney could not get any runners to volunteer for the walking part of the study at the USOTC.

Dr. Sheehan went on to speculate on how wrong the runners might be: "Runners with this attitude may well be ignoring a valuable, perhaps even essential, element in their conditioning." Dr. Sheehan's column was based on how some highly respected coaches had conditioned their athletes at the turn of the century. He specifically mentioned Harry Andrews, who coached a great runner named Alfie Shrubb. At one time Shrubb held all the world records for distances from 2 to 15 miles. "Many other runners, boxers, and cyclists of the time were followers of the Andrews method," Dr. Sheehan said. The one thing they had in common? *They all spent considerable time walking.*

According to Andrews, it did not matter whether your sport was boxing, fencing, wrestling, rowing, running, javelin, or shot put; walking as a primary exercise was applicable to all. He felt it was nature's first exercise and offered "by far the greatest benefit of any form of training in its results." Andrews's program for his budding runners consisted mostly of walking, interspersed with occasional running. Even as these athletes progressed, Andrews continued a policy of morning and evening walks. Running was limited to the afternoon, and *the time spent walking always exceeded that spent running.*

For those interested only in fitness, Andrews recommended walking; he saw it as a superior way to reduce weight. His instructions were simple: "The best advice I can give is make your own pace—the pace, in fact, that will suit you best. This pace will almost certainly be an average of 4 miles an hour."

Somewhere between 1900, when that sage advice was given, and the late 1900s, walking was shunted aside as a useful part of an athlete's training regimen, the philosophy being that the only way to improve speed is to practice it—thus running. That is partly true, but any runner's training regimen should also include the right amount of "recovery miles." High-intensity walking could play an important role in this phase of training. Many studies have shown that when duration and intensity are increased, the injury rate for runners increases dramatically. This is not true for walkers—at any intensity level.

In an effort to reduce injuries and improve performance, there is a trend among coaches and runners to use what is known as "cross-training." As Dr. Sheehan pointed out, "Runners are now encouraged to substitute some of their running time with cycling, swimming, or weight lifting." But, he added, "when we think about alternative types of training, we should consider walking, the primary cross-training activity of the early 1900's." Dr. Sheehan concluded, "It is possible that walking will enhance our running more than any of our current alternative sports." His hunch is on the money. The problem, however, is how do you convince runners, coaches, exercise physiologists, and athletes in other sports to try an innovative training mix of high-intensity walking and running?

According to Dr. Sheehan, Coach Andrews, whose athletes included cyclists, did not permit his runners to cycle as part of their training. In fact, the world record holder Shrubb warned runners against cycling, saying that it tends to "chop" the stride. Whether cycling "chops" the stride or not, world-class cyclists or swimmers cannot transfer their aerobic capacity to running the way the U.S. and Mexican race-walkers did in the USOTC high-intensity walking protocol.

In an earlier chapter, I cited a study in which trained swimmers who were tested on a treadmill running test showed *no* aerobic improvement when running. If there is no aerobic cross-training effect between swimming and running, then why is swimming recommended sometimes as a cross-training exercise for runners and high-intensity walking is not?

Dr. Sheehan had no idea what was under way at the USOTC when he wrote the closing sentence of his column: "I hope our exercise physiologists will take it upon themselves to demonstrate scientifically what the great Harry Andrews found in practice: Walking and running are no more than two forms of the same activity."

The study by Drs. Byrnes and Kearney demonstrated scientifically that high-intensity walkers not only achieved maximum oxygen uptakes similar to those of runners but also could switch to running and achieve the same oxygen uptakes without cross-training. The significance of this aberration in the specificity principle is enormous. High-intensity walking should now play a major role in a wide variety of sports and athletic aerobic-conditioning regimens, especially during rehab from sports-related injuries. Indeed, where walking has previously been universally excluded from intense aerobic training, we should find that more walking and less running will produce better athletes *with fewer injuries.*

There are unlimited physical conditioning possibilities with high-intensity aerobic walking. Let's look at a few hypothetical training regimens for a variety of athletic circumstances.

HIGH-INTENSITY AEROBIC WALKING WILL HELP RUNNERS

In the days of Harry Andrews and Alfie Shrubb, aerobic conditioning, interval training, and cross-training were unknown. Highly sophisticated equipment to test athletic fitness didn't exist. Much of what was done by coaches and athletes was done by feel and instinct. By today's standards, it was the Stone Age of exercise physiology.

Nevertheless, those early coaches and athletes must have instinctively understood that their approach helped reduce injuries, the bane of all runners. Reintroducing walking—specifically high-intensity aerobic walking—into runners' training schedules would produce two major benefits: it would reduce injuries, and it would help athletes maintain a high aerobic level by converting a large share of "junk miles" (which simply burn calories and keep body fat down) to aerobic walking miles to take advantage of walking's unique capacity to transfer aerobic fitness to running. The ultimate reduction of impact on the musculoskeletal system would be impressive.

A look at some conservative theoretical numbers will reveal just how impressive. In *Exercise Physiology,* for convenient comparisons and evaluations of body build and composition, a "reference man and reference woman" were developed. These are theoretical models based on average physical dimensions. The reference man is 20 to 24 years old and weighs 154 pounds. The reference woman is in the same age range and weighs 125 pounds.

For a theoretical runner's training schedule, let's assume that the reference man currently runs 40 miles a week, including interval training. If half of this (20 miles) was converted to high-intensity aerobic walking, what would be the reduction of impact to his musculoskeletal system in one week with no sacrifice to aerobic conditioning?

The average runner hits the ground at 3.50 times his or her body weight. A walker loads his weight onto his foot at 1.25 to 1.50 times his body weight. Any analysis of the two gaits should also take into account the way the foot makes contact with the ground. A runner is airborne, and his heel strikes the ground, introducing shock to the musculoskeletal system. By contrast, a walker is always in contact with the ground, and his heel is placed on it without impact. That is significant. A runner on each step will hit the ground with a force at least two more times his body weight than a walker's (3.50 − 1.50 = 2).

Because of running's horizontal springing action, as a rule runners take fewer strides per mile than walkers. Since we are using hypothetical numbers, let's assume that our reference man has a 4-foot running stride, which means he would take 1,320 steps per mile (5,280 feet ÷ 4 = 1,320) Pulling all the numbers together looks like this:

2 × 154 pounds = 308 extra running-impact pounds per step over walking

308 × 1,320 steps = 406,560 extra running-impact pounds per mile over walking

406,506 × 20 miles = 8,131,200 extra running-impact pounds per week over walking

By converting half of his running time to aerobic walking, the runner in the example would have reduced the trauma he puts onto his musculoskeletal system by 8,131,200 pounds in just one week.

It stands to reason that over the many years of a runner's racing career (usually starting in high school), this magnitude of impact reduction would be a significant contributor to injury prevention. Indeed, high-intensity aerobic walking could not only contribute to injury prevention in runners but could very well extend some running careers. It is probably the most overlooked and least understood training option available to runners. Creative coaches should get their runners out of the swimming pools, off the stationary exercycles, and out on the road or track doing high-intensity walking.

Alfie Shrubb may have been more observant than modern-day coaches when he also said that cycling "chops" the stride of runners. Watch the action of the leg muscles, particularly the hamstrings, on a cyclist. They never get fully extended in a full rotation of the pedals. The hamstrings were biomechanically engineered over millions of years of evolution to function for walking and running, not cycling. Getting those muscles ready for running by cycling is counter to the specificity principle. Studies by coaches and exercise physiologists should be conducted to determine whether runners (and other athletes) who train with stationary cycles suffer more pulled hamstrings than those who don't.

Now that it is proven high-intensity walking can contribute to the aerobic capacity of a runner, doesn't it follow that if runners start to train with high-intensity walking, some of them will get very good at it? This could lead to an obvious biathlon, a walk/run, in which the athlete must excel in his or her two natural gaits. This would be a challenging athletic event.

TIGER WOODS COULD BE EVEN BETTER

From a pure application of the specificity principle, perhaps no group of athletes could get more out of high-intensity aerobic walking than the professional golfers on the PGA and LPGA tours. It would do for them what no other exercise can. Until I started researching *Walking*, I had no idea that these highly paid professional athletes are still in the dark ages when it comes to proper conditioning for one of the most grueling physical and mental challenges in all of professional sports.

Why do so many professional golfers in their forties stop winning big tournaments and some young shooters fresh out of nowhere start knocking them off? Practically all professional golfers relentlessly practice driving, chipping, and putting, but few spend any time conditioning their walking gait, which must carry them through a long tournament. And young legs will beat tired older legs every time, in just about every sport.

The PGA and LPGA have highly equipped, well-staffed fitness training vehicles that follow their tours. When researching the first edition of *Walking*, I spoke with an exercise physiologist who had worked the fitness vehicle for the LPGA tour for three years and was currently working the PGA tour. He told me that there were about 150 male golfers on the tour at that time, and that each round of golf requires the golfer to be on his feet for four or five hours constantly, without ever sitting down. The same is true for the women.

The exercise physiologist explained that a typical four-day tournament is usually preceded by a one-day pro-am round, which often lasts longer than five hours. What kind of physical conditioning do the golfers engage in for this grueling schedule? Practically *none* that would contribute to their walking gait, which has to carry them through the tournament. He said about 15 percent of the male golfers do some jogging; 3 miles several days a week was typical. On a sporadic basis, 10 percent use a stationary exercycle and about 25 percent use a stair-climbing device for cardiovascular conditioning. He also said that about two-thirds of them do some stretching and flexibility exercises.

With such a lack of proper physical conditioning of the walking gait, it was not surprising that Jack Nicklaus, a golfing legend, admitted to *USA Today* that "I just ran out of gas" when he shot a 76 on the last round of the 1991 Masters. Earlier in the tournament, on fresher legs, he had a sizzling 66. With his superior talent and a high-intensity walking program, I believe Nicklaus should have been able to win many more big tournaments. But first he had to *start* with a full tank of gas. On TV, when I watched him trudge up to the eighteenth green on the last day of the Masters, I could tell by his stride that he was leg-weary.

Pro golfers take the walking gait for granted. A younger Nicklaus only had to concentrate on perfecting his game; walking on young legs made it easy. As they age, the legs become an important factor in performance for these tournament golfers. It becomes more difficult to hold the fragile parameters of a perfect golf swing together with aging, unconditioned, fatigued leg muscles. These muscles reveal their lack of conditioning in the late rounds of a tournament when drives find the rough, sand traps seem to be in the wrong place, and putts roll past the hole.

For a tournament golfer, the subtleties of fatigue in the walking gait are deceptive and everything else is questioned when the game unravels. Just because the golfer is upright and able to trudge along, no one suspects that those unconditioned major muscle groups that contribute to posture, balance, and propulsion (an integral part of every successful golf swing) could be responsible for driving into the rough or missing easy putts. Remedies for a bad round are sought on the driving range and on the putting green instead of on the road.

Older players who still show flashes of their former brilliance are prime candidates for high-intensity aerobic walking. Younger players such as Tiger Woods and Phil Mickelson who sometimes find their game falling apart on the third or fourth day of a tournament would also find that a well-conditioned walking gait would add coordinated consistency to their game. A high-intensity walking regimen of 3 to 5 miles at least four days a week would give them a pair of legs that would carry them through a golf tournament without fatigue.

Currently, Tiger Woods is the dominant golfer on the PGA tour. I have read that he takes physical conditioning seriously and has a complete training regimen that includes some jogging. Unfortunately, jogging contributes little to his walking gait, which he uses extensively in every tournament. Woods is still walking on young legs, but I have seen him make some errant drives and miss some 6- or 8-foot putts in the late rounds of a tournament; that could be the deceptive result of leg fatigue. If Tiger Woods added high-intensity walking to his training regimen, it is possible he could be even more unbeatable. As he gets older, it would definitely keep him from running out of gas, as Jack Nicklaus did in the Masters.

Equally important, every pro golfer would find that high-intensity walking has a residual benefit that running, stationary cycles, or climbing devices don't provide. High-intensity aerobic walking makes the exerciser focus his or her mind over the entire distance of the walk. The walker has to coordinate all the major muscle groups from the neck down into one fluid, coordinated athletic move, which is exactly what a golfer does on a golf swing. It requires total concentration to maintain a fast pace, which not only produces physical toughness but heightened mental concentration.

The effectiveness of high-intensity walking for women golfers might be even greater than for men. Women are such natural walkers that not only would such training work for them, but they would likely enjoy it. Every woman I know who has taken up aerobic walking says that it elevates her energy level, mental acuity, and personal confidence. There is reason to believe that many players in both the PGA and the LPGA could possibly win tournaments more consistently if they got physically fit and mentally tough for grueling tournament play with high-intensity aerobic walking.

FOOTBALL PLAYERS: TOO BIG TO JOG

In 1986, when I was writing *Aerobic Walking,* William "The Refrigerator" Perry, the big lineman for the Chicago Bears, had burst onto the scene. He was something of an oddity at the time because of his impressive size, which was over 300 pounds. Today it seems that most NFL linemen are routinely stamped out by a 300-pound cookie cutter. Even NCAA Division I linemen at that weight are not unusual. Except for professional golfers, few athletes could use high-intensity aerobic walking better than huge football players. Many of them have had invasive knee surgery even before leaving college; the extensive use of jogging to develop aerobic conditioning causes unnecessary trauma to their musculoskeletal systems, and it probably shortens their careers.

In an earlier section of this chapter, I used Dr. Albert Behnke's reference man as a basis for age and weight in my example of how much concussion a runner puts onto his musculoskeletal system when running. In this example I will use Casey's Reference NFL Lineman. Let's assume he is 23 to 26 years old, weighs an even 300 pounds, and is going to jog 3 miles a day for twenty-eight days to establish basic aerobic fitness before going to football camp.

A review of the pounds of impact he will put on his musculoskeletal system staggers the mind. Remember that a runner hits the ground with a force that is 3.5 times his body weight. Here are the numbers:

$$300 \text{ pounds} \times 3.5 = 1{,}050 \text{ impact pounds per step}$$
$$1{,}320 \text{ steps} \times 1{,}050 = 1{,}386{,}000 \text{ impact pounds per mile}$$
$$3 \text{ miles} \times 1{,}386{,}000 = 4{,}158{,}000 \text{ impact pounds per day}$$
$$28 \text{ days} \times 4{,}158{,}000 = 116{,}424{,}000 \text{ impact pounds total}$$

The last number is the impact the lineman has subjected his musculoskeletal system to—and he hasn't even put his football pads on yet. The bigger and heavier the athlete, the more important it is to reduce the long-term cumulative effect of jogging's impact on the musculoskeletal system. There has to be a better way.

While I have used linemen in this example, valuable franchise players, such as quarterbacks Peyton Manning and Ben Roethlisberger, need aerobic walking also. These multimillion-dollar players are vital to their team's success. They must have a high degree of physical fitness to survive the pounding and fatigue that constitutes their normal working day. High-intensity aerobic walking coupled with reduced jogging miles will give them a better injury-free level of physical fitness. It will be equally effective for lineman, quarterbacks, and all other members of a football team. They can all work on their speed with short wind sprints and save their legs for the game.

FROM THE ATHLETIC FIELD TO THE BATTLEFIELD

In the winter of 1991, I was glued to the TV with the rest of the nation watching Operation Desert Storm. It renewed my interest in the physical condition of our ground troops. My interest was heightened because of a letter I had received in July 1989 from a lieutenant colonel who was director of training for the infantry.

I had contacted him by telephone after I read in *USA Today* that the army was trying to train its recruits by using aerobics classes to reduce injuries from running. He seemed somewhat flustered by the story and indicated that it was merely experimental. Not long after my call, however, the *Wall Street Journal* ran a story under the heading "And the Mess Hall's Lunch Menu Offers Spinach Quiche and Yogurt," a tongue-in-cheek poke at the army and the marines.

The story read: "Say It Ain't So—Yes, It's True: Aerobics Is Now Part of the Military's Physical Regimen." There were differing opinions about the effectiveness of aerobics in the military. An outspoken infantryman staff sergeant said, "Aerobics are for wimps, plain and simple. . . . This kind of activity does not build strong soldiers mentally and physically." A Marine Corps public-relations officer told the paper: "So many soldiers were getting hurt, the military developed an exercise program that works muscles smarter, not necessarily harder."

I wrote the lieutenant colonel a lengthy letter explaining gait efficiency and the specificity-of-training advantage that high-intensity walking has over running for the physical conditioning of an infantry soldier. I even offered to conduct a clinic for him. In his reply he said that the army encourages walking, but "it is used mainly for profiled overweight and more senior soldiers." After that cold shower, it was all downhill, with comments like "Running is more performance oriented" and "Cardiovascular benefits for normal populations are realized sooner using a running program." The comment that really got my knickers in a bunch was "Running is a more natural exercise." More natural than walking? Give me a break.

There are few instances in which a high-intensity walking program could make a better direct contribution to a specifically needed level of physical fitness than that of an infantry soldier. Forced marches and battlefield conditions require fit legs and a properly conditioned walking gait. The running gait and aerobic routines contribute little or nothing to cross-training for walking. Another reason that high-intensity walking makes sense for the military is the number of women in the services. CNN reported that there were 35,000 women in Operation Desert Storm, and again, women are sensational walkers.

With high-intensity walking, it would be much simpler to turn out a highly fit soldier, male or female, with fewer injuries. For instance, a combination of about 70 percent high-intensity aerobic walking and 30 percent jogging should significantly reduce injuries. It would produce a soldier who could not only run at the army's current standards but also walk at a level that the army and marines don't even yet comprehend. From a functional standpoint, at war or peace, the latter is more important. Any young recruit who can't do what I call the "triple nickel" (walk 5 miles in 55 minutes) shouldn't graduate from basic training. Furthermore, any senior combat officer who can't do the "triple triple" (walk 3 miles in 33 minutes) should be put out to pasture. At 68 years of age, I was still able to do both.

The foregoing was written for the first edition of *Walking* but is even more appropriate today for military training. Since the invasion of Afghanistan and Iraq the army is using more National Guard and reserve units than ever before. They are coming from civilian life and many have low fitness levels; quite a few are overweight. Aerobic walking would be beneficial for both of those circumstances without the risk of injury associated with conventional fitness running.

UNUTILIZED CROSS-TRAINING POTENTIAL

While I was writing this book a friend asked, "What could conceivably be new and exciting about walking?" Without hesitation I said, "Read Chapter 10; it could revolutionize athletic training." I believe that the study at the USOTC is more impressive for what it left unanswered than for what it demonstrated. When Dr. Byrnes was explaining the study data to me in Vancouver, he said, "This study may only be the tip of the iceberg for high-intensity walking as an athletic training aid. . . . What we need now are more scientific studies to track performance results and hopefully injury reduction and experimentation by coaches and athletes in various sports using high-intensity walking as part of their training regimen."

The last words in the study abstract—"indicates a potential cross-training effect"—should have had an explosive impact on athletic conditioning. So far it has not. Even though Drs. Byrnes and Kearney worded that premise cautiously, one only has to look at Figure 10.2 to see that the oxygen uptake was higher in every instance in the running gait for the walkers. It is highly significant that the protocol at the USOTC demonstrated high-intensity walking can transfer *all* of its oxygen uptake to running. No other exercise can do that. It is clearly a major aberration in the specificity principle that cries out for experimentation and implementation by exercise physiologists, coaches, and athletes. It opens up a wide range of new training possibilities that could lead to better athletic performance, extended athletic careers, reduction of training-induced injuries, and faster recovery of aerobic fitness after an injury.

Using hypothetical training regimens, I have boldly suggested how runners, professional golfers, football players, and the infantry and marines could benefit from high-intensity aerobic walking. In addition, Dr. George Sheehan's highly respected voice urged further study of walking as a training aid. It seems incredible to me that a protocol conducted at the prestigious United States Olympic Training Center clearly demonstrating the overall potential that high-intensity walking has to contribute to athletic training would not be readily adopted by those who would benefit the most. Applying this new revolutionary approach to athletic conditioning is long overdue, but as a German proverb says, "Old errors are more popular than new truths."

ELEVEN

Race-walking
The Unheralded Athletic Challenge

The May 31, 1991, issue of *USA Today* typified the sorry state of race-walking in this country. In San Jose, California, over three hundred race-walkers from more than thirty countries were in town for the weekend to compete in the Race Walking World Cup races (20K and 50K for men; 10K for women), which are held in different countries every two years. In terms of international significance, these races are second only to the Olympic Games for race-walking.

USA Today prides itself on covering important events in the nation and spotting trends, but its sports section, which listed major sporting events for that weekend, did not give the Race

Walking World Cup a single line of type. Most of the international race-walking champions and active world record holders were in San Jose. Many went on to compete in the 1992 Summer Olympics at Barcelona, Spain. They were the cream of the crop.

The ultimate irony of this omission occurred in the same issue of *USA Today* in their sports section. The paper reported that the latest tabulations on exercise popularity showed that "the USA's No. 1 recreational sport is walking. Total walkers: 71.4 million, up 72% since 1985." That number was more than three times the number of runners and joggers in this country. Except for the *San Jose Mercury News*, no major paper gave the World Cup any pre-race coverage. The men's 20K and women's 10K (now a 20K) were on Saturday, June 1, but ABC's *Wide World of Sports* chose instead to cover a mini-marathon, which is not even a regulation track-and-field event. In the sixteen years since that World Cup event, sports coverage hasn't improved and, except for minimal late-night TV exposure in the Olympics, race-walking remains essentially an anonymous sport.

I believe that race-walking is either ignored or subjected to ridicule as a sport for the same reason that walking has been underrated as an aerobic exercise. Since walkers don't go as fast as runners, walking has not been taken seriously as an intense exercise or as a sport. Exercise physiologists and sports reporters seem to focus on speed and don't realize that walking and running are two distinct gaits, with totally different biomechanical characteristics and degrees of difficulty.

Much of the ridicule directed at race-walking comes from the technique the walkers use to achieve their phenomenal speeds. Most sportswriters and commentators who make lame attempts at humor about the technique don't have a clue as to how the biomechanics of the walking gait works. They probably don't know much about the biomechanics of the running gait, either, but assume that since it is faster, it must be a greater athletic challenge. That is not true, however, which indicates that their coverage is as shallow as their knowledge. What is it about race-walking that makes it the least understood of all the track-and-field events? Let's take a look.

RACE-WALKING EXPLAINED

Chapter 5 covered the correct posture for *all* walkers from the slowest to the fastest. Chapter 6 introduced aerobic walking with the bent-arm swing so you could increase your arm swing to match your increased stride frequency as you pick up the pace of your walk. At this point you are already two-thirds of the way to becoming a race-walker. Learning the lower body movements is the last third and the cause of much comment.

First, let me disqualify myself as a race-walking expert. I am an avid race-walking fan, however, and through my research and contacts have access to expert information. For this race-walking section I had the advice and counsel of Leonard Jansen, who was head of computer services at the Sports Science Division of the USOTC. As an analyst at their biomechanics lab, he has viewed and analyzed miles of film and videotape of the internationally ranked race-walkers. Before leaving the USOTC he was the foremost authority in the United States on the technique of world-class race-walking.

Essentially, what race-walkers do with their lower body is flex the pelvis forward as their non-weight-bearing leg swings out in front of them toward heel plant. As the pelvis reaches maximum forward flexion, it tilts down, lowering the body's center of mass as the heel is placed on the ground. This simple biomechanical maneuver accomplishes two things: (1) it lengthens the walker's stride; (2) it lowers the body's center of mass to reduce the rising and falling of the body on each step, so the walker can achieve more efficient forward progression.

As Dr. Inman explained in his analysis of the human walking gait, which was cited in Chapter 5, each walker has some natural pelvic rotation on the non-weight-bearing side of the forward swinging leg. He also pointed out that this rotation increases with walking speed. Race-walkers intentionally increase their forward pelvic flexion to bring the hip joint of the swinging leg farther forward, contributing to increased stride length.

As the pelvis is being flexed forward, it is also developing what Dr. Inman called a "pelvic list." It is tilted down away from the weight-bearing leg; thus the body's hypothetical center of mass (located in the pelvis) is lowered. In his analysis of this phase of the walking gait, Dr. Inman states: "As the walking speed increases, there is a progressive increase in the amount of drop of the pelvis to the side of the leg in the swing phase." He adds, "At higher speeds, the pelvis is not lifted all the way to a level position during the latter part of the swing phase." Race-walkers utilize this unique biomechanical feature to reduce the normal vertical rising and falling of the body, which are counterproductive for forward progression.

The forward flexion of the pelvis and the subsequent downward pelvic list create an unusual visual effect that is not associated with regular walking. Sadly, this necessary biomechanical action causes sportswriters and commentators to make inane remarks about it. They often stereotype it as a side-to-side wiggle, which it is not. The pelvic action I described may sound relatively simple, but putting it into practice along with the other subtleties and nuances of the race-walking technique requires years of training before a walker can reach top competitive speeds.

To get a quick idea of how the pelvis flexes forward and lists at the same time, stand with both feet under you, knees fully straightened and locked. Keeping one knee straightened and locked, snap the other knee forward and watch your hip on that side quickly flex forward and tilt down. While you are standing with both feet on the ground, rotate your pelvis forward and backward a few times. As your pelvis flexes forward, you can observe about how much it would contribute to your stride length if you were doing this movement in conjunction with your leg swing.

Now that you understand the biomechanics of how the walking stride is efficiently lengthened for race-walking, take a few extra long steps the conventional way, by simply swinging your legs farther out in front. You will quickly notice that there is an unrhythmic rising and falling of your body. Lengthening the stride this way would not make for an enjoyable walk and would certainly not allow you to increase your speed. The only way to lengthen stride and increase speed in a fluid, rhythmic manner is the way race-walkers do it.

The forward flexion of the pelvis also enables the race-walker to achieve inline foot placement. This virtually eliminates lateral sway of the upper body, which affects speed. It also lessens strain on the groin muscles at racing speeds. Normal walking leaves two parallel tracks, as shown in Figure 11.1A. As you learned in Chapter 5, people who track wide when they walk have noticeable lateral upper-body sway. Race walkers minimize this by walking with a single track, shown in Figure 11.1B.

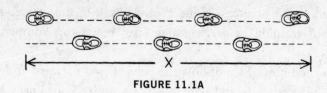

FIGURE 11.1A

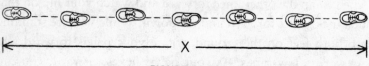

FIGURE 11.1B

To give you a better idea of the pelvis's role in this biomechanical maneuver, Figure 11.2A shows a cutaway top view of the pelvis in a normal walking stride. The feet land in parallel tracks, and the pelvis is squared to the line of travel. Figure 11.2B shows the forward flexion of a race-walker's pelvis on the right side with both feet landing in line. If this illustration could be shown in three dimensions, it would also reveal that the right hip is lower than the left. With the trailing foot almost directly behind the center of mass (see black square), and with the center of mass also lower, race-walkers can maximize forward thrust and minimize vertical oscillation of the body. Thus they are able to walk with exceptional speed.

Jansen, who also coached our World Cup team, points out that the faster times of today's walkers probably result from a changed emphasis on stride length. He explained that in years past the walker reached as far forward as possible with the swing leg. At heel plant, when the body is momentarily in the double-stance phase, the legs formed a near-isosceles triangle (having two equal sides), as shown in Figure 11.3A. Note that

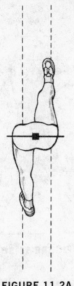

FIGURE 11.2A

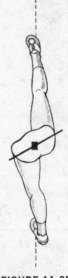

FIGURE 11.2B

the lines from the center of mass down the legs to the front foot and back foot are roughly equal. Each foot is also equidistant from the vertical line of gravity at the center of mass.

Figure 11.3B shows the new style, in which the front foot is placed closer to the line of gravity at the center of mass than the trailing foot. This position permits the heel to be planted quickly and smoothly. More important, it reduces the time that the leg is in front of the center of mass (when it is a resistance to forward progression) and increases the time that the foot is behind the walker pushing against the ground for forward thrust. The complex biomechanics of the race-walking technique are far more involved than meets the untrained eye.

The way race-walkers plant their heels and load their weight onto their feet is also important. When the swing leg reaches its

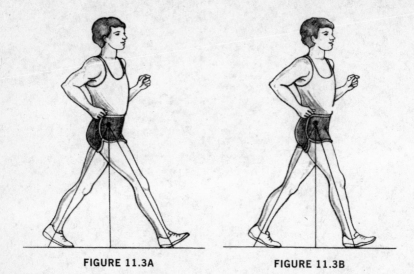

FIGURE 11.3A   **FIGURE 11.3B**

maximum forward extension, it must be straight at the knee with the toes up at a comfortable angle. As the foot is lowered to the ground, it rolls forward along the outside edge, to the ball of the foot, to toe-off (see Figure 11.4). The leg must remain straight at the knee from heel plant through the vertical weight-bearing phase.

Chapter 6 recommended that aerobic walkers place their feet on the ground with a slight emphasis on the outside edge. Race-walkers, by contrast, come down on the outside edges of their feet in a fairly pronounced manner when they load their weight onto their feet. To do this properly requires coaching and a lot of practice. I recommend that you do not attempt to walk with this abnormal foot placement without proper coaching. You will not like it, you won't be able to walk any faster, and you might injure yourself.

A race-walker leans slightly forward from the ankles; the

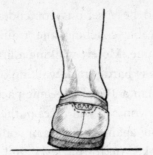

FIGURE 11.4

back is straight from the ankles to the ears, never bent at the waist. Utilizing the bent-arm swing in combination with pelvic flexion and listing, the walker develops a smooth, rhythmic, coordinated move. The pelvis should flex back and forth on each step with no side-to-side wiggle.

As each leg swings forward under the body, it should be bent at the knee just enough for the toes to clear the ground. The heel of the front foot should land directly in line with the toe of the back foot. A properly coached and trained race-walker literally skims across the ground, with every biomechanical move of the arms, hips, legs, and feet carefully coordinated to produce a highly efficient, rhythmic, fluid, forward progression. All the major muscle groups in the legs and pelvic area are used to power the walker along at phenomenal speeds. Race-walking requires the flexibility of a gymnast, the grace of a dancer, and the endurance of a marathon runner. I believe it requires more mental and physical discipline and more coordinated athletic ability to become a world-class race-walker than to become a world-class runner.

It should now be apparent why I separate race-walking from

exercise-walking. To be a serious contender in a competitive field takes considerable coaching and training to master the race-walking technique. Merely walking a little faster than normal with bent arms is hardly race-walking. Good race-walkers walk much faster than a 10-minute-mile pace. However, if you are an older person, you can win races in the 10- to 12-minute-mile range competing against walkers in your age bracket. Aerobic walking will take you to this level, and you won't have to learn the complex lower-body movements of race-walking. Using only the aerobic walking technique, I was still able to walk in that time range at 70.

RACE-WALKING RULES

Race-walking is a judged event and governed by a set of rules. The most important is Race Walking Rule 232, listed in the 2005 competition rules from USA Track and Field. It states: "Definition of Race Walking: Race Walking is a progression of steps so taken that the walker makes contact with the ground so that no visible (to the human eye) loss of contact occurs. The advancing leg must be straightened (i.e., not bent at the knee) from the moment of first contact with the ground until the leg is in the vertical upright position." You can see that the right leg of the walker in Figure 11.5 is in compliance with Rule 232.

Observe the right leg of the walker in Figure 11.6A. It is bent through the entire step cycle, which is illegal in a race. The walker in Figure 11.6B is also illegal because of loss of contact (see bracket).

In a judged race, a walker can be disqualified (DQ) if he or she receives three DQ cards from three different judges. In a road race, depending on the size and layout of the course, there

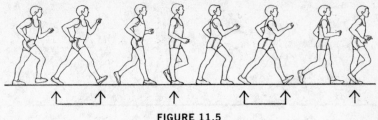

FIGURE 11.5

should be a minimum of six to a maximum of nine judges including the chief judge. In track races, indoors and outdoors, there should be five judges including the chief judge. A "runner" (usually on a bicycle or motorbike for road races) circulates among the judges and picks up DQ cards.

Each judge has a yellow paddle with the symbol for the bent leg (creeping) on one side and for loss of contact (lifting) on the other. The paddle is flashed at the walker if one of those infractions are committed and a red DQ card is sent to a DQ status board. If a walker receives three DQ cards during the race, the head judge finds the athlete on the course as soon as possible. He or she holds a red flag in front of the walker to disqualify the contestant and says something like "Number seventy-eight, Jack Jones, you have been disqualified. Please remove your number and leave the course." Judging is an important part of race-walking, and unfortunately there is a national shortage of judges.

It is my belief that Rule 232 is a major contributor to the criticism race-walking receives from sportscasters and sports writers. The loss-of-contact provision, where both feet must make contact with the ground (see brackets in Figure 11.5), is violated constantly by top walkers: because they are moving so fast, the toe of the back foot leaves the ground momentarily before grav-

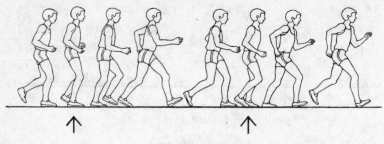

FIGURE 11.6A

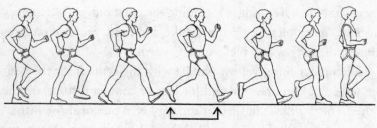

FIGURE 11.6B

ity can pull the heel of the lead foot to the ground. In race-walking parlance this is referred to as "lifting," but I believe it is more appropriate to call it "floating."

The double-contact rule has been in effect for decades; long before technological monitoring such as stop-action video was available. Ground-level cameras can detect the momentary period of float that is in violation of Rule 232. Thus race-walking is criticized for violating its own rules because the camera can see what is not visible "to the human eye." The momentary loss of contact does not help the walker go faster; it simply makes him or her in violation of Rule 232 and eligible to be disqualified. What a shame!

I have a picture of a trotting horse in the middle of a race, and all four feet are off of the ground. It is in a period of momentary float because the horse is moving so fast gravity can't pull two of its feet to the ground before the other two leave the ground. At normal trotting speed a horse (and all quadrupeds) have two feet in contact with the ground (i.e., left front/right rear and vice versa). When a horse is running there is also a moment when all four feet are off of the ground, but it is easy to distinguish visually between a trotting and running horse because the gaits are so biomechanically different. When trotting at the speed of a running horse, however, this 1,000-pound animal's horizontal momentum momentarily overrides the pull of gravity and the camera catches all four feet off the ground—but it is *not* running.

A race-walker, walking at the speed of a fast runner, experiences the same horizontal momentary float as the racing trotting horse. As a personal experiment, try to have loss of double contact on your next walk. You will find that at normal walking speeds, your front foot is always pulled to the ground by gravity before the toe of your back foot leaves the ground. Only at extreme race-walking speeds does momentary loss of contact occur, but like the trotting horse, the walker is not running.

In effect, Rule 232 requires a race-walker to put the heel of his or her lead foot on the ground faster than the pull of gravity, but that is not possible. No free-falling body or object (in this case the walker's heel) can reach the ground faster than the speed governed by the laws of gravity. If the horizontal momentum of a 154-pound walker or a 1,000-pound horse is such that it momentarily overrides the pull of gravity, then loss of contact will occur—but only for a fraction of a second. *Most important: this phenomenon does not confer a racing advantage to either the walker or the horse and therefore it is irrelevant.*

The elimination of the double-contact provision in Rule 232

would silence those who criticize race-walking for breaking its own rules. The judges would then only have to focus on whether the walker's leg had a straight knee from "the moment of first contact with the ground until the leg is in the vertical upright position." This provision eliminates any possibility the walker could cheat by running. I don't believe race-walking will gain the respect it so richly deserves until the double-contact provision of Rule 232 is repealed.

CHINESE AND RUSSIANS DOMINATE RACE-WALKING

In international race-walking competition no U.S. walkers, male or female, are listed in the top fifty rankings (based on personal best time) for 2005—the last year ranked as this was written. In the grueling 50K (31.1 miles), which is about 5 miles farther than a marathon, the Chinese held seven of the top ten positions and the Russians held the other three. The fastest time, 3:36:06, was recorded by Chaohong Yu of China. Converting his time into miles per minute, Yu *walked* the 31.1 miles averaging 6.9-minute miles. The fiftieth walker was also Chinese, with a time of 3:55:35, averaging 7.5-minute miles. Other countries in the top fifty included Spain, Mexico, Italy, France, Belarus, Poland, Japan, Slovakia, Australia, and Norway—but not the United States. Our fastest walker was timed at 4:09:35.

The 20K (12.4 miles) is the other international race-walking event and is held for men and women. In the men's 20K the Chinese captured twenty-three of the top fifty positions and the Russians took eight. The fastest time was 1:17:33, by Nathan Deakes of Australia, with a Chinese walker only eight seconds slower. Deakes walked the 12.4 miles with a blistering 6.2-minutes-per-mile average. Most of the other countries from the

50K were represented in the 20K rankings, plus two walkers from tiny Ecuador. Jefferson Perez from Ecuador had a personal-best time only 1 minute and 2 seconds slower than Deakes.

In the women's 20K the Chinese and Russian dominance continued but was more evenly distributed. The Chinese held twenty positions of the top fifty, and the Russians captured fifteen. The fastest time, 1:25:41, was by Oliampida Ivanova of Russia, who averaged a stunning 6.9 minutes per mile. The number two walker, also a Russian, was only 47 seconds slower. Among the women, Lithuania, Greece, Czech Republic, Portugal, Belarus, Spain, Germany, Ukraine, Kazakhstan, Rumania, Australia, and Italy were represented—but where was the United States? Our fastest walker was 2 minutes and 6 seconds slower than the 1:31:23 time by a Lithuanian walker who was ranked fiftieth.

Most people aren't aware of the phenomenal times these athletes walk over such demanding distances, especially the 50K. As a matter of national pride, it pains me that the United States, which has the best nutrition and most sophisticated training equipment in the world, can't produce athletes who can beat walkers from less fortunate small countries such as Ecuador, Rumania, Lithuania, and some of the others. Race-walking isn't taken seriously in this country, but that is not the case in China and Russia. The Chinese are serious global competitors in business and manufacturing, and now they even dominate a little-known sport such as international race-walking. We are so enamored of highly paid professional athletes that we don't give an amateur sport such as race-walking enough attention. To be competitive on an international level, race-walking needs more young people to take up the sport. Unfortunately, there is no feeder system for race-walking. It is not a high school track-and-field event; consequently, it is not an NCAA university and college sport. Because it is poorly understood and often unfairly maligned, many young boys and girls who would like to give it a try refrain from fear of ridicule. I hope that someday this will change.

Many track-and-field events in the Olympics are made up of arbitrarily devised physical challenges—for example, the triple jump, pole vault, shot put, discus, javelin, high jump, and hurdles. I don't believe any of the foregoing are as athletically demanding as walking at a 7-minute-mile pace for 31.1 miles. In every event there are degrees of athletic difficulty, but few can match that required by a race-walker. If track-and-field competition is analyzed on the degree of athletic ability required, race-walking should be one of the premier events.

HOW TO GET IN TOUCH

With millions of exercise-walkers out there, some are going to want to find out how fast they can walk in competition, just as many of the runners wanted to find out how fast they could race. When *Walking* was first published I listed some race-walking newsletters as a way to get information on race-walking clubs and where to find coaches and races. Some of those publications are no longer in existence, and a few are still being written by walkers almost as old as me, so their future is limited.

Now with the Internet, all you have to do is contact the North American Race Walking Foundation (www.members.aol.com/RWNARF). On that website, under the able direction of Elaine Ward, you can find clubs in your area, coaching information, and where races are being held. You can also just Google "race-walking" or "race-walking newsletters," which will give

FIGURE 11.7
ATHLETIC ACHIEVEMENTS OF FAN BENNO-CARIS

World Records

World Record 2004   3,000 meter racewalk, women 85–89   27:14 (Outdoor)

World Record 2004   3,000 meter racewalk, women 85–89   27:11:02 (Indoor)

American Record 2003   5,000 meter racewalk, women Age 85–89   42:20

World Record 2003   3,000 meter racewalk, women Age 85–89   27:30

World Record 1992   1.0 mile racewalk, women Age 70–74   10:14

World Event Results

Gold Medal   10,000 meter racewalk, women 85–89, WMA Carolina, Puerto Rico 2003

Gold Medal   5,000 meter racewalk, women 85–89, WMA Carolina, Puerto Rico 2003

you plenty of up-to-date options for race-walking coaching and races to choose from. Many older walkers who would like to learn race-walking and compete at a relatively modest level can find the information they need on the Internet. And don't think you are ever too old to learn the sport. At one of my aerobic walking clinics at the Cooper Aerobics Center in Dallas I taught Fan Benno-Caris the basics when she was 70 years old. She got hooked on the sport and went on to compete nationally and internationally in her age bracket. Among a few of her victories is the World Record in 1992 for the 1.0-mile race-walk (women age 70–74) in the sparkling time of 10:14. In other races at the world level she won gold medals in the 10K and 5K race-walks (women 85–89) at Puerto Rico in 2003. In 2004 she set two world records in the 3K (women 85–89) in 27.14 (outdoors) and 27.11 (indoors). She also has two American records confirmed for women age 85–89: 5K in 42:20 and 3K in 27:30. In a personal note to me, Fan Benno-Caris said she turned 88 in February 2006 and is *teaching* race-walking. Way to go, girl!

At any age, there is nothing that you can do better athletically to challenge your competitive spirit in a noninjurious way and at the same time improve your daily functional mobility. The walking gait is fundamental to the scheme of life for the human species and race-walking lets you take it to its highest level. Go for it!

TWELVE

Applied Exercise-walking: Medical Applications and Aging

MEDICAL APPLICATIONS

Although this book is primarily focused on walking for fitness and weight control, there are a number of diseases and rehabilitative procedures—such as cardiac rehabilitation, hypertension, stroke, type II diabetes, arthritis, and loss of functional mobility from aging—that respond best when exercise is part of the treatment. Those who have the normal function of their walking gait and any of the foregoing problems will find that walking is an ideal exercise to aid in treatment or rehabilitation. Its intensity levels can be easily regulated, for the level of exercise appropriate for each person's physical condition. *Caveat: exercise infor-*

mation in this chapter (and throughout the book) should only be implemented with the permission of your physician.

Cardiac Rehabilitation

My cardiac rehabilitation started in May 1999 when I had my near brush with death, and I continue practicing a strict rehab regimen to this day. The will to live a long healthy life is a great motivator for me. Unfortunately, cardiac rehabilitation is not as widely practiced as you might think.

The September 2005 issue of the *Johns Hopkins Medical Letter* states, "Only 10% to 20% of the eligible participants enroll in cardiac rehabilitation programs." The medical letter advises educating yourself about your condition and how to manage it, paying close attention to nutrition, exercise, and weight management, and seeking counseling if necessary. Once you have had properly supervised instruction on the essentials, adapting them as a permanent part of your lifestyle is imperative.

The more you know about "cardiac rehab," the better you will feel, physically and mentally. Obviously exercise is a critical component of cardiac rehabilitation, and in *The Cooper Clinic Cardiac Rehabilitation Program* (Simon & Schuster, 1990), Dr. Larry W. Gibbons and Dr. Neil Gordon examine the pros and cons of exercise choices. They conclude, "Most experts, including ourselves, consider walking the most appropriate aerobic activity for coronary artery disease patients." Walking is appropriate because its intensity is easy to control, so even those in the high-risk category can walk and get the desired conditioning effect. They cite another reason: "It is one of the least likely to cause musculoskeletal problems." As our primary gait of locomotion, walking is virtually injury-free.

Many patients have spectacular recoveries from heart attacks or heart surgery and become aggressive exercisers because they want to develop a maximum level of cardiovascular fitness. All too often these exercisers have been advised to use walking for their entry-level rehabilitation but to seek higher exercise intensity with running, cycling, or some other exercise as their physical condition improves. Aerobic walking as described in Chapter 6 will give anyone the fitness of a runner without risk of injury. In addition, heart patients will get the specificity-of-training effect from walking that helps them function better in their normal daily life. As Dr. Gordon said to me, "Anyone can derive *all* of their health and fitness needs from a walking program."

As of this writing, cardiac rehab following a heart attack is covered by Medicare, and many private insurers will cover at least part of the costs. If you don't have access to a rehab center, your doctor can recommend some exercises that are suitable for your health situation and level of fitness. It takes *you*, however, to make the commitment to rehab the most important muscle in your body—your heart.

Hypertension

Hypertension (high blood pressure) is the most common cardiovascular disease, affecting about 58 million Americans, with more than half having some degree of heart-related involvement. More than 60,000 deaths a year are attributable to hypertension and hypertensive heart disease. The December 2005 issue of the *Mayo Clinic Health Letter* states, "Even a healthy person with normal blood pressure at age 55 has a 90 percent lifetime risk of eventually developing hypertension." This is a warning that all the baby boomers should heed. It adds, "Simple lifestyle choices—such as what you choose to eat, how active you are and reducing excess weight can influence your blood pressure and long-term health."

Exercise-walking can be effective in controlling mild hypertension without medication in some cases, or it may be used in conjunction with medication. Dr. Neil Gordon recommends an aerobic intensity of 60 to 85 percent of the maximal heart rate. He says that exercise duration and frequency should be regulated so that about 1,000 to 2,000 calories a week are expended. Many people who engage in this level of exercise are ultimately able to discontinue high blood pressure medication. However, if you are also trying to lose weight at the same time, you will need considerably more caloric expenditure, which you can achieve through walking.

Stroke

It is not commonly known, but stroke is the third leading cause of death in the United States, after heart disease and cancer. A stroke is a potentially fatal cutoff of the blood supply to part of the brain. When the blood supply to any part of the brain is reduced, the oxygen-starved cells in that area stop functioning properly. For those who survive a stroke and whose rehabilitation program has brought them to a stage at which only a slight to moderate disability remains, a regular exercise program will help increase functional capacity and lessen the chance of having another stroke.

In his book *Stroke: Exercising Your Options*, Dr. Gordon warns: "Stroke is a *recurrent* disease, and if you've had one stroke you are five times more likely to have others. To put it another way, of the 62 percent of people who survive a stroke, about one quarter can expect to have a second stroke unless they do something to prevent it." This is one of the primary reasons he believes that you should start exercising once your formal stroke rehabilitation program is over—that is, if you can. Not every stroke survivor recovers enough to be able to exercise regularly.

Dr. Gordon writes: "Moderate exertion several days a week is likely to greatly reduce the chances that you'll develop a second stroke or die prematurely from other various potentially chronic diseases." Just as important, exercise will help reduce your disability. Even though you may have to walk with a slight limp caused by irreversible neurologic impairment, you may be able to increase the frequency and distance you can walk, which reduces your degree of disability. If you are a stroke survivor who is lucky enough to still have a good, functioning walking gait, use it for all it's worth. It may be your ticket to a longer, healthier life.

Type II Diabetes

Type II diabetes (formerly called adult-onset diabetes) is a complicated disease that has become a full-blown national epidemic since *Walking* was first published in 1992. Its medical dangers and costs were the subject of an editorial titled "Declare War on Diabetes" in the *New York Times* on February 5, 2006. The editorial stated that in New York City alone, one in eight adults has diabetes, which is almost 150 percent higher than ten years ago. On the front page of the same issue the *Times* chronicled the lives of the oldest living diabetics, Gerald Cleveland, 90, and his brother, Robert, 85. During their lives the Clevelands suffered some medical complications and close calls, but as the *Times* reported, "The Clevelands have lived long and healthy lives in part through extraordinary discipline in diet and exercise."

The May 2005 issue of the *Johns Hopkins Medical Letter* states that people with type II diabetes must improve their nutrition and exercise levels in order to keep their glucose levels under control. The Clevelands are long-living proof of that advice. One of the reasons people develop type II diabetes is that their cells have grown resistant or insensitive to the insulin circulating in the blood. Exercise improves insulin sensitivity and is essential for weight loss.

The obesity problem sweeping the country is a major contributor to type II diabetes. Weight loss increases insulin sensitivity, which in turn improves blood glucose control. Getting weight down into the ideal range is often the only treatment that type II diabetic patients need to normalize their blood glucose levels. Exercise-walking is the most effective, sustainable exercise for weight control, and it is particularly effective for someone with type II diabetes. However, there are precautions to take before starting an exercise program.

The Mayo Clinic website (www.mayoclinic.com) advises, "Be sure to talk to your doctor first if you've been inactive and plan to start a program of regular exercise to manage your diabetes. He or she can tell you about any precautions you need to take and likely conduct a pre-exercise physical that focuses on your: 1. Heart and blood vessels, 2. Eyes, 3. Kidneys, 4. Blood supply to your legs and feet, 5. Nervous system, 6. Blood pressure." Type II diabetes affects so many parts of the body that a pre-exercise physical can help spot potential problems.

A diabetic should be extra cautious about getting blisters

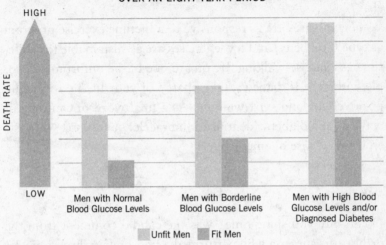

FIGURE 12.1

STUDY INVOLVING 8,118 MALE COOPER CLINIC PATIENTS
OVER AN EIGHT-YEAR PERIOD

DEATH RATE — HIGH ... LOW

Men with Normal
Blood Glucose Levels

Men with Borderline
Blood Glucose Levels

Men with High Blood
Glucose Levels and/or
Diagnosed Diabetes

Unfit Men   Fit Men

Source: Neil F. Gordon, Diabetes: Exercising Your Options. Champaign, IL: Human Kinetics Publishers, in press.

from shoes or socks, because reduced blood flow to the feet affects the healing process. Formfitting socks, preferably a synthetic blend to wick the moisture away and keep the feet dry, are a must, as are properly fitted shoes. Before putting your socks on, check your feet for blisters or areas of redness where a blister may be starting to form. You may want to put a Band-Aid or some gel on the affected area. Follow the same procedure after exercise. Even without type II diabetes an exercise-walker can't function well with blisters, and a diabetic can't function at all. Be careful!

Exercise-walking will make you fit, which is a major plus for a diabetic. Figure 12.1 shows that fit men with high blood glucose and/or diabetes had about the same death rate as unfit men with normal blood-glucose levels. Fit men with borderline blood glucose actually did better than the unfit men with normal levels.

Few diseases are as responsive to a lifetime exercise program as type II diabetes, and few exercises are as sustainable for a lifetime as exercise-walking. If you are one of the unfortunate people with type II diabetes, take charge of your life in a forceful, positive way and start walking. As a final word of caution, always wear a diabetic identification bracelet or shoe tag while exercising, in case of emergency.

Arthritis

"I can buy you some time" was the candid comment from the orthopedic surgeon who performed a two-hour arthroscopic debridement on my right knee in January 1987. It was the third operation on the knee since 1973, and the advanced osteoarthritis was evident in the X-rays even to my untrained eye. Arthritis finally prevailed, and my "time" ran out in May 1995, when I had to have a total knee replacement. Arthritis wasn't finished with me, and the other knee was replaced in August 2004. Maintaining an aggressive walking program over the years that arthritis was doing its damage wasn't easy. Some days were more painful than others, but every exercise day contributed to my overall health and sense of well-being. Now, thanks to the miracle of modern medicine, I complete my daily walks pain-free.

The word *arthritis* is derived from two Greek words, *arthron,* "joint," and *itis,* "inflammation." Literally, it means "inflammation of the joint," and those who have it (or had it, as in my case) can certainly attest to this. Osteoarthritis has the distinction of being the oldest and most prevalent chronic disease known to humans, and for most types of arthritis there is no known cure. Damage is limited to the musculoskeletal system, usually in weight-bearing joints—feet, knees, hips, and spine. However, it also invades the joints of the fingers, hands, and toes and also the shoulder, neck, back, and elbow.

Until recently, experts thought osteoarthritis resulted from normal wear and tear on joints, but current thinking is that a variety of factors are responsible. In his book, *Arthritis: Exercising Your Options* (Human Kinetics Publishers, 1992), Dr. Neil Gordon writes: "Aging, repetitive impact on the body's weight-bearing joints, genetics, and some other as yet unknown biochemical processes are responsible for osteoarthritis." Baby boomers who are turning 60 in 2006 and all those who follow should be aware that almost half of all Americans 65 years or older have some debilitating arthritic condition. Even about 28 percent of Americans between 45 and 64 years old have some form of arthritis.

For centuries, rest was viewed as the only way to alleviate arthritis. Even gentle exercise was considered harmful. This has all changed, and for several decades doctors have been prescribing stretching exercises because they help to preserve joint function. While rest helps reduce joint inflammation, excessive rest is deleterious. In only one week of immobilization, a muscle can lose about 30 percent of its bulk. Dr. Gordon points out that recent evidence indicates that aerobic exercise can aid in arthritis rehabilitation.

Supporting that observation was a study published in the April 2005 issue of *Arthritis & Rheumatism,* which indicated that vigorous activity cuts arthritis disabilities. The study stated, "Older persons with chronic conditions need to be encouraged to participate in physical activities, regardless of their current capabilities." More than 5,700 people at least 65 years old participated in the study, which indicated that inactivity nearly doubled the loss of physical function among seniors with arthritis.

As people age beyond 60, they tend to slow down, even if they don't have arthritis. Arthritis compounds the effects of inactivity and contributes to the wasting of muscles; weakness of muscles, ligaments, tendons, and bones; degeneration of joint cartilage; and "contractures," which reduce the range of a joint's mobility. Clearly there is reason for someone who is arthritic to exercise.

Obviously the level of an individual's arthritis determines what exercises are appropriate. Dr. Gordon says, "The preferred exercises are low-impact aerobics such as walking, cycling, and swimming." Your doctor's consultation is advised to determine if a weight-bearing exercise such as walking would be beneficial. People with advanced osteoarthritis may find more tolerable, sustainable exercise in the buoyancy of a swimming pool. In addition to the exercises mentioned, Dr. Gordon states: "*Daily range-of-motion exercises for the affected joints are absolutely essential*" (emphasis in original). A gentle yoga program is a way to accomplish this.

During my personal bout of osteoarthritis while my knees were deteriorating, there were many times I could have decided not to walk, but I feared that might cause me more overall harm. Arthritis inflammation ebbs and flows—some days are better than others. A little aspirin and a couple of days off now and then bought me some relatively pain-free walking. Don't throw in the towel if you have arthritis. Inactivity and lack of exercise can be your worst enemies. Pick an exercise you can tolerate in relation to your arthritic condition and go for it. If exercise-walking is tolerable, you will find it contributes enormously to your fitness, functional mobility, mental attitude, weight control, and sense of well-being.

AGING AND WALKING

Like a pig through a python, the baby boomer generation is creating a big bulge in our aging population as the first wave turns 60 in 2006. In articles in magazines and newspapers and in feature segments on TV, many boomers indicate that turning 50 means they are "old." Even worse, some imply that the good life is almost over. From my 79-year-old perch up here on the longevity spectrum, being 50 would make me feel like I was a teenager again. Believe me, people who hit the half-century mark and adopt a healthy lifestyle have some of the best years of their life ahead of them. As the late Joe Frisco, a popular comedian of the thirties and forties, once said, "You only live once, but if you work it right, once is enough."

Whether you are younger or older than a baby boomer, it is interesting to see how various age ranges perceive how old is "old." In July 2005, WebMD reported a Zogby International survey conducted for the MetLife Mature Market Institute that asked the participants "How old is 'old,' and how old are you?" Nearly a third of the participants thought someone 71 to 80 years old was "old." Those under 30 used the "old" label for those 61 to 70. And people who were at least 65 said "old" meant being 71 to 90 years old.

This survey closely parallels one that appeared in the AARP's magazine, *Modern Maturity,* in which people under 30 thought 63 was old, and those over 65 thought 75 was old. The common denominator in both surveys is that as people age they keep moving their perception of "old" farther up the longevity scale. When I was under 30 I also thought anyone in their 60s or higher was old. Now I really am old and I don't have any room to move the perception of "old."

Old age must be viewed from two perspectives. One is the chronology of our years, and we all age equally in this category. Second, but more important, is biological aging and one's functional activity level. My energy level and physical condition now in many respects are better than when I was 45, sedentary, and 52 pounds heavier. I saw this same disparity in almost every one of my walking clinics. Highly active 70-year-olds and even some 80-year-olds outperformed sedentary 50- and 60-year-olds. Although they were older in years, their eyes were brighter, their step was quicker, their balance was better, their energy level was higher, and their outlook on life was more upbeat. What gave them this edge when chronologically they were 20 years older? Exercise!

In a poll on longevity conducted by Charlton Research for *Parade* magazine and Research!America in 2005, under the heading "Factors in Aging," the question was asked: "How important do you think each of the following factors is in how well a person ages?" (Figure 12.2A). In a triple tie at 85 percent, physical activity, diet and nutrition, and mental activity were rated *very* important.

In another poll, the question was asked: "What one thing, more than any other, makes you think of a person as being 'young'?" (See Figure 12.2B.) The response of "Active/energetic/busy" was first at 50 percent and equaled all other responses combined. In fifth position was "Age" at only 3 percent. Baby boomers and all others who think age is what makes them appear "young" should take heart and start exercising; that is the

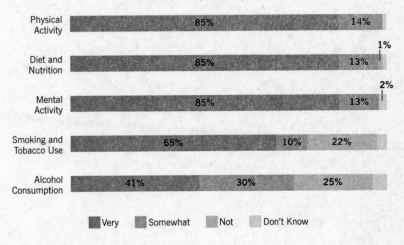

FIGURE 12.2A
FACTORS IN AGING
How important do you think each of the following factors is in how well a person ages?

Source: *Longevity Poll, 2005—Charlton Research Company for Research!America.*

major contributor to remaining active and energetic, and it is definitely associated with being "young" beyond your years.

"What Americans Think About Aging and Health" was the headline of *Parade*'s story on the latest poll in their February 5, 2006 issue. The lead question was: "Thinking about the prospect of living to a very old age, what one thing would you worry about the most?" (See Figure 12.2C.) Rated first by a large margin at 37 percent, the respondents said, "Poor, declining, failing health." In a press release from Research!America preceding the story, Lee Kravitz, editor-in-chief of *Parade,* said, "Americans have concerns about aging and health, but they have an even stronger belief that healthy aging is possible with preventative steps like exercise and a healthy diet." He is ab-

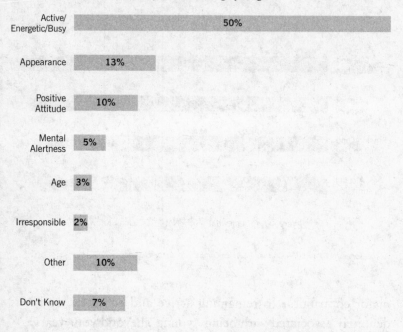

FIGURE 12.2B

BEING ACTIVE AND ENERGETIC ASSOCIATED WITH BEING "YOUNG"

What one thing, more than any other, makes you think
of a person as being "young"?

- Active/Energetic/Busy — 50%
- Appearance — 13%
- Positive Attitude — 10%
- Mental Alertness — 5%
- Age — 3%
- Irresponsible — 2%
- Other — 10%
- Don't Know — 7%

Source: Taking Our Pulse: The PARADE/Research!America Health Poll—Charlton Research Company, 2005.

solutely right. Adopting a healthy lifestyle with exercise and eating smart are the best steps anyone can take for healthy aging.

As people age, the range of exercises they can and should do narrows considerably. As a longtime avid exerciser, I am a living example of that. I am walking as hard as I did fifteen years ago, but my pace is slower. It takes longer to warm up, and my range of motion in some joints is not the same. I keep walking every day, however, for my health and because it is well established

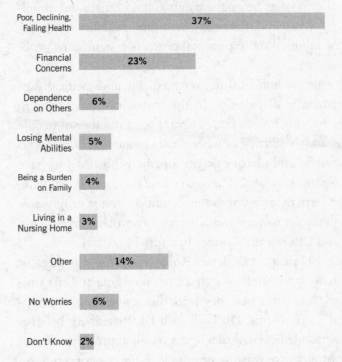

FIGURE 12.2C

HEALTH IS A #1 CONCERN

Thinking about the prospect of living to a very old age,
what one thing would you worry about most?

Poor, Declining, Failing Health	37%
Financial Concerns	23%
Dependence on Others	6%
Losing Mental Abilities	5%
Being a Burden on Family	4%
Living in a Nursing Home	3%
Other	14%
No Worries	6%
Don't Know	2%

Source: Taking Our Pulse: The PARADE/Research!America Health Poll—Charlton Research Company, 2005.

that if you want to maintain a skill or function you must use it. The more we do something the better we are able to do it. Playing a piano or using a computer are obvious examples of that.

A more important example is walking, which we all seem to take for granted. I have some older friends who have had to give up driving a car. Depending on your age, that may seem like a huge sacrifice, but it is a minor annoyance compared to not being able to walk. More than any other activity or exercise, walking (because of the specificity principle) conditions the older exerciser so that he or she can maintain functional mobility to carry out normal, necessary activities. Inability to simply take care of minimal daily personal needs is a significant problem as people age.

As a hospice volunteer, I deliver medicine and medical supplies to terminally ill patients. In that capacity I have been in most of the nursing homes in this area. I see a number of people in their 60s and 70s sitting in wheelchairs in nursing homes who have no specific ambulatory or orthopedic problems but have simply ceased to function. They have lost their ability to walk. Perhaps the term that describes this condition best is *progressive wasting of muscle tissue,* which I learned from Dr. Steven Blair, president and CEO of the Cooper Institute in Dallas.

Dr. Blair told me that Dr. Irwin Rosenberg, who was director of the Human Nutrition Research Center on Aging at Tufts University, used this term when they were discussing the aging population and its problems. Dr. Blair said Dr. Rosenberg believes this is a serious medical disorder and a national problem. He believes that progressive wasting of muscle tissue is a condition requiring study and definition and that ultimately it should be given a medical name (as happened with the well-known term *osteoporosis*). Drs. Blair and Rosenberg think many people can halt or reverse the wasting of muscle tissue by becoming active again. There is ample evidence to support their position.

In 1991 Dr. Rosenberg and William J. Evans, another Tufts University professor, wrote the then revolutionary book *Biomarkers: The 10 Determinants of Aging You Can Control.* In the book they addressed the progressive wasting of muscle tissue and called it *sarcopenia.* If you Google *sarcopenia* you can get a detailed explanation of the term. The main message of *Bio-markers* remains as true today as in 1991; "Exercise is the key to a healthy and rewarding old age."

Fast-forward to May 2006 and in a special supplement to the Tufts University *Health & Nutrition Letter,* Dr. Rosenberg, who is now the editor of the newsletter, revisits the premise of *Bio-markers.* The *Letter* states that with exercise and good nutrition you can slow down the loss of strength and decrease in metabolism; postpone conditions such as heart disease and osteoporosis; and stop the onset of *sarcopenia,* a weakening of the body's muscles, particularly in the legs, with a loss of muscle mass and replacement by fat. The ultimate price of this condition is loss of balance, reduced mobility and the frailty so often seen in the elderly."

The *University of California at Berkeley Wellness Letter* reported that many experts estimate that half the functional losses that set in between the ages of 30 and 70 are attributable to lack of exercise. When aging is accompanied by inactivity, it can result in declines on the following scales: "(1) Muscle fiber is lost at the rate of 3–5% a decade after age 30, leading to a 30% loss of muscle power by the age of 60; (2) By middle age, blood vessels typically narrow by 29%. Between the ages of 25 and 60, the circulation of blood from arms to legs slows down by as much as 60% and (3) The speed at which messages travel from the brain to the nerve endings decreases 10–15% by the age of 70." Although the foregoing occurs with inactivity and aging, regular exercise has been shown to inhibit, arrest, or even reverse such declines. It is time for you to take stock of your age and your exercise program (if you have one) to see if you are doing all that is necessary to help stall the biological aging process.

To arrest the progressive wasting of muscle tissue requires

adding weight training to your exercise regimen. I have experienced muscle loss of the quadriceps (front thigh muscles) since my knees were replaced. Those muscles used to be large and well developed, but after the operations they atrophied. Even though I do weekly leg lifts with my Bowflex machine I have never been able to regain the size and strength they once had. Arm and chest muscles also tend to wither as we age, and require weight-training exercises. YMCAs and health clubs have instructors qualified to guide you in a weight-lifting routine if you can't afford to buy your own equipment. The object is not to bulk up but to tone up. I can tell you from personal experience, the older you get, the more you need it. Don't delay in getting started.

As stated earlier, the major muscle groups in the body are located below the waist. They are the walking muscles. By engaging in an aggressive exercise-walking program you stop the progressive wasting of muscle tissue, increase your functional mobility, and contribute to your overall health. You can stall biological aging! Sadly, however, as people age they tend to walk less, not more. And the less they walk the less they are able to walk.

Many of the elderly (and I am one) curtail their walking for fear of falling. As Dr. Inman points out in *Human Walking*, walking is not a reflex action but a neural process and must be learned.

When learning to walk, very young children fall many times but get up and try again and again until they finally learn how to walk. An 80-year-old who falls while trying to relearn how to walk may never get up again. For many elderly people, the fear of falling is one of their greatest terrors. Falls are the sixth leading cause of death in the elderly, and a fractured hip is among the most common and debilitating health problems that older people face. My fairly healthy 93-year-old mother passed away nine days after fracturing her hip.

Where there's a will there's a way, and not only can older people be retaught how to walk, the results can be spectacular and they enjoy it. When the first edition of *Walking* was being written, an exercise program for extremely elderly people was being conducted at Heartland Regional Medical Center's health facility here in St. Joseph. It was called Walk to Washington and involved seventeen people (fifteen women and two men) with an average age of 85. One of the women walkers was 101 years old. The program started at 11 a.m. and quickly became the focal point of their day. In three months they accumulated 170 miles, which is the equivalent of walking across the state of Missouri from St. Joseph to Hannibal.

Most of the walkers, especially several who were recovering from fractured hips, started out tentatively. Some walked looking down at their feet. The longest distance covered in a day by a walker was four city blocks and the shortest only 100 feet, but to every participant it was an accomplishment of which he or she was proud. The hospital staff reported that all of them had better appetites and better morale. They were more animated and slept better because even this small amount of mobility widened their horizons. Everything in life is relevant, right up to our last breath.

Baby boomers and those who are at an advanced age, let the specificity principle be your overriding guide for exercise. Exercise-walking, more than any other exercise, contributes to your balance, agility, and functional mobility. All three are essential as you age.

Unfortunately, as many people age, their inactivity increases, and they reach what Dr. Blair calls a "functional disability threshold." They lose mobility to the extent that they don't have the physical capacity to take care of such simple personal needs as going to the grocery store. At this point nursing homes become an unwelcome alternative for many of them. Inactivity is a compounding, debilitating cycle, and within nursing homes people often develop an inactivity threshold in which they are not even mobile enough to walk to the bathroom or to the dining room. It can happen to anyone who doesn't have a fit, functioning, walking gait.

The primary health goal for all who are 60 or older is to maintain an exercise and activity level that can extend their ability to remain independent and mobile. Dr. Neil Gordon calls the loss of independent living "compressed morbidity," and Figure 12.3 demonstrates this loss of functionality. For the aging population walking combined with stretching and flexibility exercises constitutes the perfect exercise combination. Exercise-walking's intensity can be gentle, moderate, or vigorous to accommodate all levels of fitness. Unlike most other exercises, walking contributes directly to the all-important aspect of functional mobility.

After studying the compressed-morbidity chart in Figure 12.3, I have decided on the way I would like to go to the hereafter. If Dr. Gordon will move that bottom dot over to 100, when my time comes I want to *walk* down to the undertaker and expire on his doorstep. A tough old walker might as well save the pickup fee.

Figure 12.3 shows theoretical curves for two individuals. The line labeled "independent living" indicates a threshold of function required for living independently. When a person's functional capability falls below this threshold, he or she must be institutionalized or receive custodial care. In this example,

FIGURE 12.3
COMPRESSED MORBIDITY

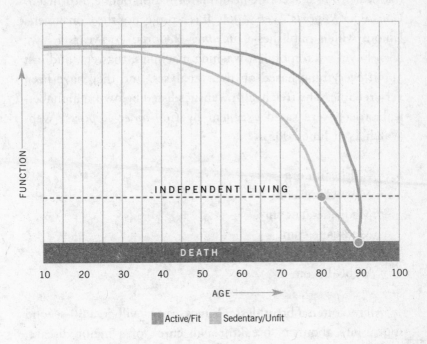

Source: *Institute for Aerobics Research*, The Strength Connection.

both people die at age 90. The sedentary person had to be institutionalized for the last ten years of life. The active person can
live independently until near the end of life—a worthy goal we
all should try to achieve.

STAYING CURRENT

Ubiquitous Internet access has made free medical information
available to everyone with just the click of a mouse. Not all on-

line health information is reliable, however, and some can be harmful. To find accurate health information online, I turned to *Consumer Reports*' WebWatch. It is a project of the Consumers' Union, which publishes *Consumer Reports*. For years I have been buying automobiles, washing machines, toasters, and just about everything based on their analyses, and they have been very reliable. The free health websites listed below (in alphabetical order) were rated excellent by *Consumer Reports*' Web-Watch as of June 2005.

- Kidshealth.org
- MayoClinic.com
- MedicineNet.com
- Medscape.com
- National Institutes of Health (www.nih.gov)
- WebMD.com

All too often a breathless TV newscaster will do a 30-second sound bite about a "breakthrough cure" of a major disease, when medically it hasn't progressed beyond mouse studies and a "cure" is years away, if ever. If you have gotten your hopes up with this kind of vacuous information, go to one of the recommended websites for the complete, reliable story. The breadth, depth, and quality of free health information available today are unparalleled. At any age, two of the most important things a person can do are to stay informed about health-related matters and to exercise. The information is free and so is the exercise.

THIRTEEN

Mental Aspects of Walking

It is not commonly known, but the walking gait can work its magic from the neck up as well as from the neck down. The least publicized application of exercise is the role that it plays in the management of mental stress, depression, anxiety, and mental acuity. Exercise is generally emphasized for weight control and cardiovascular fitness, but it will also relieve tensions, elevate self-esteem, dissipate hostilities, and build self-confidence. Like aspirin, exercise is a generic medicine and has a wide range of applications. There are many exercises and all of them have some merit, but the walking gait is unrivaled for its physical and mental contributions to our well-being.

In our sedentary lifestyle, the human body, both physically and mentally, is starved for exercise or for some form of regular physical activity. The Greek physician Hippocrates, who is called the father of medicine, said, "All parts of the body which have a function, if used in moderation and exercised in labours in which each is accustomed, become thereby healthy, well developed and age more slowly, but if unused and left idle, they become liable to disease, defective in growth and age quickly." Hippocrates made that observation about 2,400 years ago. His words are even more relevant today.

As you contemplate the role of exercise in your life, heed Hippocrates's words that all parts of the body that have a function should be "exercised in labours in which each is accustomed." Walking fits his description perfectly. In the animal kingdom, our upright walking gait makes us unique, and we are biomechanically engineered to be walkers. No exercise machine or arbitrarily designed physical fitness routine can duplicate the all-encompassing beneficial effects that a good walk will contribute to our total well-being. Our body is its own self-contained exercise machine, which needs to be put in motion.

MENTAL PROBLEMS

Under the heading "Walking: Big Benefits for the Brain," the September 2005 issue of *The Johns Hopkins Medical Letter* reported on two separate studies published in the *Journal of the American Medical Association* that suggest walking regularly may help preserve mental sharpness. The medical letter stated, "In a study of more than 18,000 female nurses age 70 and older, those who walked the most (at least 1.5 hours per week) scored higher on tests of general thinking ability, verbal memory, and attention than did women who walked the least (less than 40 minutes per week)." In addition, the most active women were 20 percent less likely to be considered cognitively impaired.

In the other study, walking's mental benefits were evident on the male gender, showing that in a study of more than 2,000 men over 70 years old in Hawaii, walking on a consistent basis slowed down the onset of dementia. Researchers suspect that better overall cardiovascular health—which translates into improved blood flow to the heart and brain—is behind the better mental functioning of the exercisers. Research also suggests that exercise promotes the preservation of brain cells and increases the connections between them.

The November 2005 issue of the *AARP Bulletin* reported a study from the Karolinska Institute in Sweden, conducted on 1,500 people ages 65 to 79. They found that those who engaged in robust physical activity at least twice a week since youth or middle age had a 50 percent lower chance of developing dementia and a 60 percent lower risk of developing Alzheimer's than those who were sedentary. As the article pointed out, "Swedish participants who reduced their odds for dementia engaged in aerobic exercise." That type of aerobic activity works the large muscle groups in the legs, arms, and hips. It also raises the level of oxygen in the blood and increases the heart rate over a sustained period (of at least 20 minutes). Aerobic walking fits this description perfectly.

The idea that regular exercise can help your head as well as your heart and joints was supported by Dr. Walter Bortz, clinical associate professor of medicine at Stanford University in the same *AARP Bulletin* article. He said, "What's good for the knee is good for the neurons. When you do biceps curls with weights in a gym, blood and oxygen go to the biceps muscle and it enlarges." And he added, "Same with the brain when you run or walk or do other forms of aerobic exercise. You're getting more blood and oxygen to it."

DEPRESSION

Among the many mental disorders in this hectic world, depression and anxiety affect a wide range of people of all ages. A study titled "Prospective Study of Physical Activity and Depressive Symptoms in Middle-aged Women" was conducted at the University of Queensland in Brisbane, Australia, and reported in the November 2005 *American Journal of Preventative Medicine*. This study examined the dose-response relationships between self-reported physical activity and depressive symptoms from a population-based group of middle-aged women who participated in the Australian Longitudinal Study on Women's Health between 1996 and 2001. The study showed a direct correlation between an increased physical activity and decreased depressive symptoms in middle-aged women.

Between 1998 and 2001 the Cooper Institute, Behavioral Science Research Center in Golden, Colorado, conducted a study titled "Exercise Treatment for Depression: Efficacy and Dose Response" that was reported in the January 2005 *American Journal of Preventative Medicine*. It was designed to test whether exercise is an efficacious treatment for mild to moderate major depressive disorder (MDD) and the dose-response relation of exercise and reduction in depressive symptoms. All exercise was performed in a supervised laboratory setting with adults of both sexes age 20 to 45 diagnosed with mild to moderate MDD. The participants were randomly assigned to one of four aerobic exercise treatment groups that varied total energy expenditure and frequency consistent with public health recommendations for physical activity. At the public health recommended level, aerobic exercise can help treat mild to moderate levels of MDD. Any exercise at a lower level is comparable to the placebo effect.

WALKING MEDITATION

The foregoing studies indicate that exercise, especially aerobic exercise, can have a salutary effect on a number of mental disorders. As Dr. Bortz indicated, what works for the heart also works for the mind. As someone who is at high risk for a heart attack and a follower of Dr. Dean Ornish's approach to cardiac care, I have found that in addition to physical activity, quiet time in the form of meditation also benefits the heart and mind. The March 2005 *Mayo Clinic Health Letter* reported on the body-mind connection in an article on meditation. It stated, "Meditation is a mind-body process—when focused, the mind is calmed and the body can relax, creating a sense of well-being. The mind's health influences the body's health."

According to the National Center for Complementary and Alternative Medicine (part of the National Institutes of Health), "regular meditation can improve longevity and quality of life. It can also reduce: 1. High blood pressure, 2. Anxiety, 3. Substance abuse, 4. A hormone (cortisol) in the blood stream that increases with stress, 5. Post-traumatic stress syndrome, and 6. Visits to a health care provider." The health letter advised that, "Meditation alone doesn't replace medical treatment. But it does appear to reduce stress and may positively influence the effect of more standard treatments."

Some forms of meditation are easier to learn than others.

Among the various forms, mindfulness meditation is growing in use in the health care field. Being mindful means you are able to pay attention to your experience from one moment to the next without being carried away by other thoughts or concerns. I learned the mindfulness meditation technique from Dr. Jon Kabat-Zinn's book *Full Catastrophe Living* (Dell, 1990), which I mentioned in an earlier chapter when I recommended yoga. I use Dr. Kabat-Zinn's yoga tapes. He also considers yoga a form of meditation.

Sitting meditation is the frequently practiced form of meditation and the one I use the most. However, Dr. Kabat-Zinn also has a chapter in his book on walking meditation, and it is very effective. It further demonstrates the versatility of our walking gait. Dr. Kabat-Zinn says, "Walking meditation involves intentionally attending to the experience of walking itself. It involves focusing on the sensations in your feet or legs or, alternatively, feeling your whole body moving. You can also integrate awareness of your breathing with the experience of walking."

He further advises, "To begin walking as a formal meditation practice, you should make the specific intention to do it for a period of time, say ten minutes, in a place where you can walk slowly back and forth. Since it looks weird to other people to walk back and forth without any apparent purpose, especially if you are doing it slowly, you should do it someplace where you will not be observed, such as your bedroom or living room." I use the long hall in our house, which is perfect for walking meditation. To be effective, sitting meditation is best done in a private, secluded setting also, so don't be self-conscious about walking back and forth slowly in absolute privacy.

Up until now I have focused on the benefits of a faster-paced walk, but with walking meditation, the slower the pace, the better. Dr. Kabat-Zinn says, "To deepen our concentration, we do not look around at the sights, but keep our gaze focused in front of us. We also don't look down at our feet. They know how to walk quite well on their own. It is an internal observation that is being cultivated, just the felt sensation of walking, nothing more. Mindful walking can be just as profound a meditation practice as sitting or doing the body scan or the yoga." I was in my early 70s and quite skeptical when I first attempted yoga and meditation. Both take learning, concentration, and commitment, but once you have embraced them, the benefits to your mind and body become obvious. I am living proof that you really can teach an old dog new tricks.

A NATURAL TRANQUILIZER

Family, marital, financial, and health problems are some of the major sources of stress that are pervasive in our society today. If you are experiencing mental stress from problems in your life, take your troubled mind for a long walk to smooth out the wrinkles in your psyche. A daily walk is nature's catharsis for the emotional strains that seep into our lives. It is the analgesic for life's pain and the antidote for life's poisons. Walking, preferably outside, will take you back, physically and mentally, to life's natural pace. It will let you cut the mechanical and electrical umbilical cords of the machines and screens that connect you to the modern world (so please don't forget to turn off your cell phone).

The intensity of your walk will tend to match your level of stress. Anger, for instance, will often succumb to a fast pace. I have never started a walk angry and ended up the with same feeling I had when I began. You can literally walk your anger into the ground. As troubled thoughts flow in and out, let your mood set the pace of your walk and guide you into a tranquil state of mind. At the risk of sounding redundant about the many physical and mental health benefits of exercise-walking, there is one aspect that does need repeating, only because it is so difficult to get people to believe it: it makes you feel good. Without exception, all the exercise-walkers I know say that they sleep better at night and that they have a higher energy level during the day, greater self-confidence, better mental acuity, and a more positive outlook on life—*plus they feel good!*

THE COMPLETE EXERCISE

Walking is a universal elixir for the body, mind, and spirit. You will find that it is nearly impossible to walk daily in the outdoors without engaging in spiritual introspection. If you are able to walk in rural areas, as I do, and observe the beauty of nature, you will find that the mind tends to seek a higher meaning to existence than this brief journey we call life. You may find that in addition to its physical and mental benefits, a daily walk can also be a time of spiritual fulfillment. Some walkers tell me they commune with their Creator as they walk under the beautiful sky dome of His magnificent outdoor cathedral, with its ever-changing tapestry of cloud shapes and varied hues.

To conclude on a high note, I have searched in vain for something other than the overused cliché "can't see the forest for the trees." Unfortunately, that better than any other choice of words describes many people's quest for an exercise or exercise machine that is physiologically more beneficial than walking. Starting with a slow 30-minute-per-mile stroll, down to a fast race-walking pace of 6 or 7 minutes per mile, the walking gait provides an unparalleled range of injury-free exercise and athletic challenge. In the forest of exercises and exercise machines, walking is the tallest tree of all; it truly is the complete exercise.

We must part now, but I hope this book will motivate you to start walking for your body, mind, and spirit. Perhaps our paths will cross someday and we can share a walk together. In the meantime, I wish you good health and a long, happy life.

Acknowledgments

The thought of updating and rewriting my walking book at the tender age of 79 seemed overwhelming. Thankfully, the generous help of good friends turned it into a mentally rewarding experience. Dr. Kenneth Cooper, who has inspired my dedication to a healthy lifestyle for over two decades, graciously wrote the introduction. Some of my other friends at the Cooper Aerobics Center lent their support. Dr. Tedd Mitchell provided medical and exercise advice when needed, and Kathy Duran-Thal, nutritionist at the Cooper Wellness Program, shared her information on healthy eating.

My dear friend Dr. Ann Thorne led me through the intricacies of AppleWorks on my trusty iMac; I affectionately dubbed her my ghost nerd. Steve Wenger of Heartland Regional Medical Center made his lifestyle charts and medical research files readily available. Sandy Jacob's quick fingers did most of the transcribing.

I am probably alive today to write this update thanks to my good friend Bob Fay, who responded to my urgent call about my heart problem and expeditiously arranged the angiogram that I wrote about in the preface.

My longtime friends Dolph and Barbara Bridgewater gave me encouragement and the gentle nudge necessary for me to tackle the project.

A number of fine people in medicine, exercise, and science were very generous in supplying me with their research material, sharing their knowledge, and even critiquing various chapters for me to make sure my manuscript was correct in the first edition. That information is included in this edition and my heartfelt thanks go to Drs. Neil Gordon, Steven Blair, John Duncan, William Byrnes, Jay T. Kearney, and Professors Owen Lovejoy and R. McNeill Alexander. I am extremely grateful also to the late Dr. George Sheehan for writing the foreword.

Finally, Laura Ford, my editor, who happens to be a runner and over a half century younger than me, patiently persuaded me to modify the tone of the book. Her editing mellowed my comments and molded my exercise advice so that it would be motivational and appealing to exercisers of all ages. Thank you, Laura!

Index

CASEY MEYERS is a retired businessman who found a second career as an exercise-walking expert after the 1987 publication of his first book, *Aerobic Walking*. Since then, he has conducted hundreds of lectures and walking clinics across the country, including regular walking clinics for the Cooper Wellness Program at Dr. Kenneth Cooper's Aerobics Center in Dallas, Texas. He is 79 years old and walks three miles daily with his wife, Carol, and two dogs in St. Joseph, Missouri.